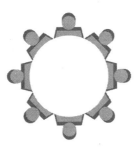

HELPING YOURSELF & OTHERS

The training manual for practitioners in the helping professions, students, clients, and all persons wishing to increase their personal insight and self-awareness.

RICHARD KNIGHT

ISBN 978-0-9524392-1-9

Printed and bound in the United Kingdom

Typeset in Tahoma

Helping Yourself and Others:
The training manual for practitioners in the helping professions, students, clients, and all persons wishing to increase their personal insight, self-awareness, and interpersonal skills

Published by
Cross Roads Publications,
16 South Primrose Hill,
Chelmsford,
Essex,
CM1 2RG
UK

t. 07966174466

A Thought Shared

"...having now travelled in many directions and tried my hand at numerous things, I have arrived at the point where my heart is telling me to focus my energies on helping others.

You see, I've been occupied with other matters although more recently I've been establishing closer links with different people and different ideas.

I know helping others begins from where I am...own motivations, intentions, and desire to be genuine. I do believe I have much to give and much to receive and wish now to develop a fuller understanding.

I'm conscious of that vital desire for the door to open further to new possibilities – possibilities which endeavour to penetrate the shrinking and expanding nature of my own and others behaviours and experience.

I know of course, and am not wishing to deceive you, that I live daily with the knowledge of my own imperfection. Once I would be concerned if my opinions were unduly influenced by the facts but now my mind is more welcoming of the generosity of different conclusions, theories, and actions, which aim to unify rather than separate..."

Table of Contents

TO THE READER
A Thought Shared

Foreword

CHAPTER ONE: **What is Helping?**

CHAPTER TWO: **The Learning Environment**

CHAPTER THREE: **Exploring Our Inner World**

CHAPTER FOUR: <u>**Considering a Practical Theoretical Framework**</u>

CHAPTER FIVE: <u>**Am I Going Mad?**</u>

CHAPTER SIX: <u>**Discovering Others**</u>

CHAPTER SEVEN: <u>**Contracts and the Management of Time**</u>

CHAPTER EIGHT: <u>**Being with the Helpee**</u>

Handout One:	Client-Centred Helping and Counselling Skills: Summary of Process, the Core Skills, and Principles
Handout Two:	List of Attitudes for Discussion and Development of Own List
Handout Three:	A Values List for Discussion and Development of Own List
Handout Four:	Questions about My Interpersonal Style
Handout Five:	Statements on My Interpersonal Style
Handout Six:	Maslow's Characteristics of Self-actualized People
Handout Seven:	Maslow's Meta-values
Handout Eight:	Trait Checklist
Handout Nine:	Considering My Script and Other Questions
Handout Ten:	Exploring Thoughts and Feelings
Handout Eleven:	Further Exploration of Self

Foreword

This book is written primarily for persons involved in the broad spectrum of the helping professions. Its focus, within the context of helping, is upon that element of the helping relationship associated with interpersonal skills, interpersonal style and the counselling process. It has been long recognised that the interpersonal dimension is critical if the outcome of helping or counselling is to be successful.

The contents of the book can be utilised by all persons who are motivated toward the understanding of their own selves and their relationship with others. The fact that the material is presented to guide practitioners and those training to be practitioners will in no way discount its application for persons outside of the formal helping networks, and will be of equal value to clients.

An eclectic approach toward helping is discussed and consequently draws upon a range of sources. The material is enhanced by the author's extensive experience, not only in direct work with patients, but also in the training of professional practitioners.

Few would argue that the helping relationship is a simple one. It is rarely easy to appreciate the nuances of another's world view and behaviours – especially when discomfort is evident – physical or emotional.

Coming close to people, in order to understand them more clearly, and subsequently assist them in understanding themselves, demands experience and skill. Skill is related to the creative use of personal gifts and intuitions, the utilisation of proven knowledge and teaching, developed by many eminent authors and practitioners. Experience, of course, takes time to gain and is dependent upon an ongoing monitoring and objective analysis of one's progress.

The material which follows forms the core elements of the helping skills repertoire. Each one of us, at different points in our lives, seeks help from others and, of course, others seek help from us. Effective helping is therefore approached thoughtfully, sensitively, and with humility. Initially, the skills are probably best acquired in a training group. Many such groups operate up and down the country and provide the opportunity for the acquisition of such skills in both a didactic sense and also experientially.

The pronoun 'he' is used throughout and is to be read as including the pronoun 'she'.

The terms helper, counsellor, facilitator, therapist, teacher, carer, clinician, lecturer, are to be read as assuming similar roles and functions.

The terms client, patient, helpee, learners, student, are to be read as being interchangeable. (With regard to these terms, they embrace all persons participating in their own study, training, therapy, learning, and personal development, irrespective of age, qualification, experience, or motivation and reason).

My thanks go to all the authors, teachers, helpers, and patients, who have been in part the source of my own development and learning, and I trust, at some level you will be able to make good use, for yourself, of some what is presented here.

I especially acknowledge the support received from Paul Phillips, IT Consultant regarding design and layout, Steve and Leah Ellefsen from Vivado Marketing Communications for cover design, Andrew McCulloch for proof reading, and from Valerie, Esther, Reuben, and Ramona, for being who they are. I dedicate this book to all those carers, and professional helpers, who have genuinely committed their life to the care and service of others.

Richard Knight.

Chelmsford 2011

CHAPTER ONE

What is Helping?

If helping has any meaning at all, it must be enabling people to achieve wholeness. Unless the helper himself is actively involved in developing his own wholeness, then the wish to become a helper will involve arrogance and dishonesty...by inviting others to do what the helper himself is not prepared to do. Out of respect for the helpee, helping must be approached from the position of humility. We all have needs, the person being helped and the person helping. In other words: within the helper is a client and within the helpee there is a helper. A client has strengths and an enlightened helper will recognise this fact. If this is not recognised, the client is denied the helper within himself.

As already suggested, helping is aiming, potentially, at wholeness. **The whole person is free from debilitating anxieties or psychotic tendencies having the basic needs for belonging, love and self-respect gratified. The whole person makes full use of his talents and capacities in doing the best he is capable of doing.**

Abraham Maslow (1971) summarized this idea of the whole person within his concept of self-actualization – the capacity for a human life of quality, built upon openness and awareness. He recognised that this is an ongoing process but, in contrast to many others, the self-actualizing person is aware of his imperfections, owns them, and makes choices about keeping or overcoming undesirable traits.

Change invariably involves discomfort as it is a process of giving up old behaviours and adopting new ones. Within our old behaviours we have been able to define ourselves in a certain way, for example, 'I am an angry person' – giving up angry behaviours will imply uncertainty in relation to 'what kind of person will I be without the angry behaviours?'

Everyone has their own conflicts or inadequacies in at least a number of dimensions. When a person is faced with persistent and overwhelming odds against which he has to prove his adequacy, he is likely to resort to all kinds of mechanisms, such as aggression, illness, rationalisation, and other inadequate ways of meeting life's demands. He soon finds himself in a vicious circle of having to resort to the same mechanisms with greater vigour and frequency. In time, ever greater threat is met with increased self-defence and an increasing inability to accept reality and the need for change. For example, our ambitious executive who more and more frequently resorts to alcohol as a means of coping with the risk of failure; or the troubled homemaker who in failing to deal with her own low self-esteem, or self-worth seeks some sense of security by withdrawing from the world and remaining within her home.

In summary then, **helping is providing the helpee with an enabling opportunity to explore, discover, and clarify ways of living more satisfyingly**. Effective helping demands of the helper continuing **self-monitoring and self-development.**

It is the relationship between the helper and the helpee that is the medium or channel of the entire helping process. The material of the relationship will be an interaction of attitudes, emotions, and behaviours of the helper and the helpee.

Among the key criteria associated with effective helping and therapeutic work is the notion of **acceptance,** described by Carl Rogers (1951) as follows:

'...the therapeutic phenomenon seems most likely to occur when the therapist feels, very genuinely and deeply, an attitude of acceptance of and respect for the client as he is, with the potentialities inherent in his present state. This means a respect for the attitude which the client now has and a continuing acceptance of the attitudes of the moment, whether they veer in the direction of despair, toward constructive courage, or toward a confused ambivalence. This acceptance is probably possible only for the therapist who has integrated into his own philosophy a deep conviction as to the right of the individual to self-direction and self-determination.....It may help to discuss briefly the meaning, (within this context) of the term **'respect'....respect for the person unrevealed.** It is a respect for something *underneath, an acceptance of the person as he seems to himself at that moment. It is only as he is dissatisfied with this self that he explores further into his feelings and attitudes...'*

A Code of Practice:

Any profession of worth has to operate within a framework or code that reflects its belief systems and operational principles. This is necessary in order to inform, and assure users of the given service, and also provide a structure for practitioners. In other words the purpose of a code of practice is to establish standards for helping and thereby inform and protect those persons seeking help.

Ethical standards comprise of values. Felix P Biestek's book "The Casework Relationship" (1961) is of unique importance in exploring and understanding the ethical principles contained in the helping relationship. The following code of ethics is developed from Biestek's work and is the basis from which proper and genuine professional practice should operate:

☐ human beings have the right to be treated as an individual which embraces the notion of personal difference including race, culture, age, gender, and intellectual, physical, and socio-economic position. In short, the recognition that everyone is exceptional

☐ the recognition of the helpee's right to express feelings openly as an essential part of the helping process without the helper discouraging or condemning the expression of feelings. Feelings are an integral part of the total personality and are, therefore, of vital concern to the helper and demand from him a purposeful response and a controlled emotional involvement with the helpee

☐ the acceptance of the individual as he is, with his own beliefs and values, and thereby assisting the helper to understand the helpee's perceptual framework and thus explore the helpee's problem or difficulties in a more realistic way. Each of us endeavour to conduct our lives according to our perceptions no matter how futile or misguided our behaviour may be to a person whose perceptual outlook is different

☐ helping involves the helper in making evaluative judgements about the attitudes, actions, or feelings discussed or transmitted by the helpee. As a consequence, the helper must adopt a non-judgemental attitude in the helping relationship and in doing so exclude assigning guilt or innocence to the helpee. **A non-judgemental attitude accepts the principle that each of us is in the process of 'becoming' – no one has 'become'**

☐ the helpee has the right to self-determination and freedom in making their own choices and their own decisions. The helping process directly involves the helpee in exploring his own capacity for positive and constructive decision making within the framework of his own self-determination, and

☐ the helper has the ethical obligation to preserve, with confidentiality, the personal and secret disclosures shared by the helpee. Therefore, 'treating with confidence' means not revealing any information through any public medium which could lead to the identification of the helpee

The foregoing Code of Practice clearly places the individual patient at the centre of the helping process. There are many different theoretical perspectives associated with the helping task. In this book an eclectic approach is explored with **Transactional Analysis** being the primary theoretical model. However, the actual **helping-style** recommended, and underlying all the interactions and processes discussed, is that of **client-centred therapy.** This approach was developed by Carl Rogers (1951) in the belief that **only the client has the answers to most of his problems,** and that only the client is able to find those answers given the right kind of caring environment, support, space, and time necessary to do so.

With a client-centred approach to helping the practitioner tries neither to impose change on the patient's perception of himself, nor interpret what the patient might disclose. The skilled practitioner, through his own adopted position of **unconditional positive regard** for the patient, will reflect back to the patient **empathically and congruently** that which is being presented, thus encouraging the patient to assume ownership of the problem/s, gain increased insight as to the likely causes, and hence empower the patient to make the necessary changes in their life in order to heal, grow, and 'become'.

An effective and skilled practitioner will use different skills at different times according to what seems to be most helpful. Particularly in the early stages (but also throughout the process), when the practitioner is trying to gain a clear view of what may be the problem/s, it is essential to **listen carefully to all that the patient is saying,** including their non-verbal language, and to respond to that which is being conveyed.

By listening carefully, better described as **active-listening**, and then communicating what the practitioner is hearing back to them is essential in establishing a rapport with the patient. It is important to note that there is a distinction between listening and hearing! Hearing involves the capacity to be aware of, and to receive sound. Listening involves not only receiving sound but also involves trying to accurately understand, and to mirror back an understanding of what is being expressed, to the client. As such, active listening entails: hearing words, volume, audibility, pace, enunciation, stress, monotony, high and low pitch, melodrama, change in pitch, shrillness, sombre cadence, intensity, accent, speech disturbance, being sensitive to vocal cues, changes in tone and mood, body language, as well as taking account of the circumstances or symptoms being described.

Active listening therefore is one of the primary core skills because it:

☐   creates rapport (when the client feels 'heard', safe, and understood)

☐   creates the opportunity for the helper to 'influence' the process by

☐ creating the necessary trust as well as displaying competence

☐ provides a knowledge base for the helper by 'hearing' information without questions, again demonstrating competence, and develops trust. (If the helper listens well then most clients will collaborate in providing further relevant information thus adding to the process and aims)

☐ the client feels affirmed, accepted, understood, and will talk more about the real issues of concern to him

☐ encourages ownership and personal responsibility to problem solve, and

☐ provides the client with a good model to learn from

Therefore, in summary, the application of listening skills will help clients to feel more secure enabling them to understand themselves at a deeper level, feel they are being heard with sensitivity, establish a task-orientated relationship that will then assist the patient in finding and valuing their own capacity for self-direction and change.

Client-centred work avoids the connotation that the client is 'sick'. In a very meaningful and accurate sense the experience of 'being heard' and consequently through the experience of being empowered, the actual experience of the 'therapy' becomes diagnosis, and this diagnosis is a process which goes on in the client rather than in the intellect of the clinician, who may otherwise be asking himself 'What does that statement mean, how might I interpret that comment?' In fact the question is 'How does the patient see this issue?' **(See Handout One: Client-Centred Helping and Counselling Skills: Summary of Process, the Core Skills, and Principles)**

Who Should Help?

Helping is useful only to the extent that it facilitates growth. The helper can no more help unless someone is helped than a shopkeeper can sell unless someone buys. Our knowledge is such, based upon our own experience, which no one can do our growing for us. Thus, **all growth is "self-growth"** and this fact is discussed later in this chapter.

The helper's role is partly one of stimulating and guiding the client towards attaining his own goals in the most efficient and effective way possible. Because of the importance of the helper in promoting and assisting clients in their maximum development, the question of who should help must be addressed.

Helpers are both 'born' and 'made'. It is a matter of first selecting students of ability and genuine motivation. Then providing them with knowledge of the subject of helping and the techniques by which both they and the client can attain potentially the highest degree of self-realisation. As indicated above, a dynamic interaction exists between these elements.

Of course, we must always bear in mind that helpers are human – nobody expects them to be perfect. There will always be helpers who are more effective than others. However, both society and the client, have the right to expect a certain degree of confidence from what might generically be called 'The Helping Professions'. It is those who have begun to explore, and to experience and question their own selves, who are likely to make the most perceptive and tolerant helpers.

The prospective helper will need to consider thoroughly:

☐ 'Why do I wish to become involved in the helping professions?'

☐ 'What makes me think I will make a good helper?'

☐ 'What assets, personal qualities, do I bring to the helping situation that will enable me to do an effective job?' and

☐ 'What do I consider might be the wrong reasons for wishing to help others?'

Before we address these questions, it needs to be said, that it is in the best interest of all concerned that those unsuited to helping be guided away from the profession. Having said this, it is still not easy to pinpoint the personal characteristics that make for effective helping.

In considering the qualities that are generally agreed to be necessary it is, by implication, reasonably safe to assume that those persons without such qualities would be unsuitable. So, what then are personal assets to be looked for in a potential helper – given that effectiveness is an aspect of the total person!

Experience places weight on such characteristics or assets as:

- emotional stability – someone who is secure and open to experience, is relatively free from anxiety and uses his energies positively and thereby increases his sense of security

- kindness – someone who is able to identify with his fellow human beings and wishes to contribute responsibly and unselfishly to others

- consideration – someone who realises others have needs that they are endeavouring to meet and therefore this is recognised when responding to others

- patience – someone who recognises limitations contained within situations or individuals, and allows for this accordingly

- openness – someone who is prepared to interrogate their own values or belief system in a meaningful way and is secure in doing so, and

- good disposition – someone who has a positive view of themselves, is in touch with their own feelings, and interacts with others in a warm and genuine way.

Of course, in addition to the above there is a need for professional competence, and the need to make full use of professional insight in promoting the prospective helpee's all round growth.

The suggested personal assets or qualities imply someone with understanding, or potential understanding, respect for the helpee, and someone who encourages within the helping relationship a sense of trust, and responsibility as well as professional alertness. However, no system has yet been devised that will fully identify good prospective helpers, and subjective judgements will feature in any selection process.

Selecting People for Training in Helping:

The selection process is invariably based around individual or group interviews. For an interview to be meaningful the required atmosphere is one that is relaxed so as to facilitate an open exchange of views. Discussion is likely to be initiated around the following range of questions which are most likely to 'test' the candidate's motives and assets:

☐ Why do you wish to be a helper?

☐ What do you understand to be the skills of helping?

☐ What do you understand a good interpersonal relationship to be?

☐ What particular qualities do you think you bring personally to the helping environment?

☐ Are there aspects of your own behaviour that you would wish to change?

☐ What values do you believe should inform a helping relationship?

☐ What might be the implications of environmental influences on growth?

☐   What do you understand to be the meaning of 'a whole person?'

☐   If you were interviewing people for training in helping what personal characteristics and competences might you be looking for?

The interview provides the best vehicle for ascertaining someone's suitability, relevant experience as well as their personal qualities, characteristics, and assets. In addition, the selection process will confirm:

☐   that the person concerned has a satisfactory level of understanding, aptitude and is committed to study and the acquisition of skills

☐   is able to express themselves clearly and articulate their views in a non-dogmatic way which implies an openness to different views and perceptions

☐   is an individual who projects a sense of trust and responsibility, and

☐   has an interest in, and is committed to, their own self-improvement

A major issue concerning people involved in helping is the matter of 'whose needs are they meeting?' There is a mutual dependence between the helper and the client and the helper may, consciously or unconsciously, be serving his own needs, for example, pursuing a perverse power role over a 'victim'. Sheldon Kopp (1974) in his book, 'An End to Innocence' states:

'...many personal and professional caretakers remain unconsciously focused on filling their own inner needs for care. Some have become chronic helpers out of despair of finding someone to take care of them. Now when they feel hungry they settle for feeding others...'

This is a difficult issue to resolve – indeed it would seem some people have more to give than others and there is also the altruistic element of people wishing to 'give back' for something received. The resolution must rest in the helpers' willingness to explore their own motivation, be prepared to acknowledge various unresolved issues within themselves, be prepared to spend time working on their own development, and always to recognise the reciprocity of the helping relationship. Helping is never a one-way process. It is an interaction, and therefore contains the sharing of feelings and experiences.

Moreover, the medical model where the client is seen as inadequate or diseased and the helper as healer and 'whole' must be avoided. **Change for any of us only becomes possible if we know where we are, or have been, or who we are, and where we might go.** The first step is identifying the illusions governing all our present actions. **Adaptability, toleration of uncertainty, and ambiguity are signs of good mental health.** It is not necessarily intentional that people refuse to modify their behaviour in ways which would benefit them, but they choose to cling to their present behaviours as change is threatening, difficult, and uncertain. **Being a person implies becoming a person, this notion is at the core of helping.**

It is worth reminding ourselves of the choices pertaining to the respective roles within any helping relationship:

<u>The Client has Choices:</u> in terms of whether to:

☐ discuss their concerns

☐ how much they may choose to reveal

☐ how and when to reveal it

☐ how much to trust the helper

☐ whether or not to work on specific issues or concerns

☐ choice of feelings about self and helper

☐ choice of thoughts and inner speech about self and helper

- choice as to how to behave between contact, and

- choice as to whether to have further contact

The Helper has Choices: in terms of whether to:

- help

- what to say

- how and when to say it

- what methods to adopt

- feelings about self and the helpee

- thoughts and inner speech about self and helpee

- limits set on contact with the helpee, and

- whether to continue with contact with the helpee

The Person-Centred Practitioner Believes:

- every individual has the resources to grow

- human nature is essentially social

- self-regard is a basic human need

- persons are motivated to seek truth

- perceptions determine experience and behaviour

- the individual (client) should be the primary reference point within any helping activity

- individuals should be related to as 'whole persons' who are in the process of becoming

- individuals should be treated as doing their best to grow given their current internal, and external, circumstances, and

- it is important to reject the pursuit of authority, or control, over others, and to seek to share power

Growth as a Person:

In any book about helping there will be frequent references to 'growth as a person'. This concept applies to the helper, the prospective helper, and of course the helpee, in other words, all of us. It is not simple to describe what this 'growth' implies. At the beginning of this chapter the whole person was described as someone who makes full use of his talents and capacities in doing the best he is capable of doing. Growth as a person is about building upon such criteria. **Whatever development and individual displays at any given time is the result of the interaction of environmental influences and internal responses, adaption, and choices, related to such influences.**

The inter-relatedness of the various aspects of development, for example innate potential, heredity, diet, early training experiences, physiological factors like proper maturation and functioning of the glands, psychological factors like a positive self-concept, and a readiness and openness to new ideas and options, are of major importance in considering an individual's capacity or inclination to grow. **What each of us will become is decidedly unknown. It is a question of the individual accepting his inner condition as forever changing since growth is change.**

The 'growing' individual knows what he is (as far as this is known to him) and knows that his potential self is even greater. He is open to new sensations and deeper emotional reactions and changes in thoughts and wishes. **Helper competence is about generating and facilitating a persons potential to grow.**

Any consideration of effectiveness in fulfilling the helping task must be made against the fact that change can be the only measure. A positive outcome must arise from a helpee understanding more fully what causes him to behave in a particular way.

Behaviour, whether desirable or undesirable, does not just occur as it arises in response to some form of external or internal stimulus. In other words, all behaviour is purposeful. Behaviour, therefore, occurs in response to needs. The concept of needs, drives, goals, or motivations, are the keys to understanding behaviour and as such form part of the helpers 'toolkit' and are also worthy of exploration in the selection of prospective trainees.

- **needs**: at all times each one of us has multiple needs to satisfy, eating, drinking, seeking approval, wanting material objects, satisfying career opportunities, and so on. The continued frustration in the meeting of needs leads to 'maladjustment' or disturbance in the individual as he attempts to clutch at any option that may provide a momentary relief in his attempts to satisfy needs

- **drives:** there is some ambiguity between needs and drives but it is suggested drives are the internal stimulus that direct us toward certain needs, for example, the need for affection, achievement, independence, approval, and recognition. Naturally, with regard to the idea of 'drives' is implied the notion of goals

- **goals:** individual goals will, of course, differ. Needs and drives and the achievement of goals are determined by individual motivation. Needs, drives, and goals provide the conditions for activity and the concept of motivation refers to the amount of energy, determination, or effort an individual is prepared to exert in order to satisfy such conditions

The classification of needs, drives, goals, or motivation are unavoidably arbitrary as they are interacting processes and the behaviour shown by an individual at a given point in time is not the outcome of a single factor but the result of multiple influences both internal and external.

The motivated individual orientates himself towards a goal which past experience leads him to believe will be effective from the standpoint of his motives. **Behaviour does not just happen: it is caused by some need, and is orientated towards some goals. Behaviour is, therefore, always purposive.**

Understanding, and acknowledgement, of the complexity of the determinants of human behaviour provides the practitioner and each of us, with the preconditions necessary to appreciate and then to live fully with all that goes on inside of us. And to be aware of the possibility of a deeper and meaningful contact with the world outside of us – in other words 'we become more open'.

Openness is the opposite to 'defensiveness', as a defended person hears only what he wishes to hear according to his own bias. **The defended person cannot be a growing person because horizons are closed.**

Carl Rogers (1961) points out that **when a person functions freely, their reactions can be trusted; they will be positive, forward moving, and constructive. An effective helper is such a person.**

CHAPTER TWO

The Learning Environment

To inspire learners, irrespective of age, at all levels of experience, knowledge, and qualification, to use their potential for maximum self-realisation is obviously the most important task facing the facilitator. In the final analysis, it is he who is the key to motivation and success in the classroom. He needs to help students develop personal adequacy as well as academic and practical competence – enthusiasm for study through a planned sequence of relative success in an atmosphere of psychological safety. **The essence of all that follows relates to all helping situations.**

Learning involves the reorganisation of experience into systematic and meaningful patterns of thinking, feeling, and behaving. The emphasis of learning process in on:

☐ the relationship with the subject and material being taught

☐ meaningfulness in terms of commitment and openness to what is being shared, and

☐ and clarity associated with the ideas being conveyed on the one hand and received on the other

Of much importance is the learning environment since it is that which a student is in part reacting to. The lecturer or facilitator has the responsibility for recognising the different strengths and weaknesses within any learner, or student group, and reconciling such differences so that meaningful learning is accessible to all. Both internal and external stimuli are involved in the motivation of behaviour and the learning process. As discussed in Chapter One, the determinants of human behaviour defined as needs, drives, goals, or motives are clearly activated within the learning environment.

There are two <u>Components Involved</u>:

☐ **meeting a need,** and

☐ **achieving an external goal**

The importance of these **two components cannot be overstated. They underlie every phase of human relations** and only when the facilitator is fully aware of this can he provide effective teaching and guidance to students in directing their behaviour and in reinforcing their behaviour towards the achievement of particular goals. Moreover, within the learning environment the facilitator must concern himself with such specific needs of students as:

☐ **<u>the need for affection and recognition</u>:** this involves warmth, friendliness, approval, and actually taking time out to relate to the respective student as an individual and not just part of a learning group

☐ **<u>the need for belonging</u>:** this is related to the need for affection and recognition, and has much to do with the individual, and experience from which all members of the group may benefit. The responsibility on the facilitator is to demonstrate that he is dependable and that the group is a safe place to be. In other words, there is security within the group, and

☐ **<u>the need for achievement and self-esteem</u>:** in this context it is the facilitator's responsibility to ensure that individuals are given material that will challenge their abilities and also provide an opportunity for success, a sense of failure compromises an individual's self-concept. **A meaningful learning environment provides the opportunity for the individual to explore what 'he is' and what 'he does' without suffering feelings of guilt or inadequacy**

Of course, some individuals have more difficulty in satisfying their needs than others. Yet, the facilitator must provide every learner with the opportunity to satisfy needs in an acceptable and desirable way. In recognising the mutual interdependence of the facilitator and the students, an opportunity exists for an enlightened facilitator to attempt to meet others needs in an open way within the learning situation. This will, thereby, **mirror the climate and ethos of the helping relationship.**

Learning in a Group:

The fundamental issue here is the social nature of any group. The facilitator will, in addition to subject matter, use the group to stimulate the learner into action. Such stimulation does not stem from the authority of the facilitator within the group but rather the relationship between himself, the task, and goals of the group.

The significance of group-work learning is that the group also provides, in relation to what is being taught, the opportunity for members to gain a better understanding of themselves in relation to other people. Such insight into human behaviour cannot easily be achieved as effectively in any other way. This is why group learning and helping, is so often adopted as opposed to predominantly one-to-one work.

To gain a better understanding of self, and achieving some sense of self-awareness, is not a simple process. The group provides an opportunity for self-disclosure and should become one of the mores and expectations of the group. Awareness is an emotional event and runs contrary to the popular belief that the intellect is the principle avenue of learning. Self-disclosure must, of course, be handled sensitively and the facilitator has a key and fundamental role here in terms of being a positive and effective role model.

There is a tendency among all of us to recognise problems in others and to deny them in ourselves. Anything that probes the nature of our identities can be threatening. The group provides an opportunity for students to become fully engaged in their own perceptions, behaviour, and communication patterns. The combination of experiential and didactic methods provides the most effective learning opportunities.

The aims of a learning group are summarised as follows:

- to help the learner acquire the skills necessary for the development of an effective helping relationship

- to help the learner become aware of their attitudes, and their attitudes towards others

- to learn approaches and techniques in order to facilitate meaningful interaction with others

- to help the learner become aware of the perceptions and attitudes others may hold

- to help the student learn approaches and techniques to effectively counsel others, and

- to provide the learner with the opportunity to penetrate their own experience and extract from it the essence of what they need to know

To provide students and with the opportunity to move from:

- **experience to reaction, to reflection, to conceptual understanding in order to expand their own understanding and effectiveness,** and

- **to provide students with the opportunity to make a link between their inner world and understanding, to that of their outer world life experience, and back to increased understanding of their inner world**

Since the relationship between our outer world and inner world is of crucial importance for all our decisions and choices, this relationship must be addressed in the group so that the learner has the opportunity to probe deeply into both realms. This, I suggest, can only be achieved through a combination of **experiential learning and reflection.**

The Elements of Training:

A range of material and approaches needs to be utilised. These will include: didactic learning, reading lists, reference material, lectures, seminars, experiential learning, individual work as necessary, being a helper and helpee in the group with the associated use of observation and feedback, and supervision.

A balance between cognitive and experiential parts of the programme needs to be established. If the theoretical part attempts to be all encompassing it is likely to fail. The students will fail to gain a clear and comprehensive picture of any approach, and will tend to be bewildered by a vast array of hypotheses.

Given the number of psychological hypotheses, it will only be possible for the facilitator to have time to skim the surface. It is preferable, I suggest, presenting one coherent model in detail, with less complete sketches of alternative schools of thought. It would be unrealistic to assume that one training programme could equally offer comprehensive cover of all the various psychotherapeutic models.

With the wish to have uniformly high standards the dilemma for the facilitator is how to balance accessibility to theoretical material and allow, through group experience, the student to become 'sensitised' to that material. **The value and appropriateness of what is being taught will be ascertained from two key features within any training group, these are supervision, and how the individual is experiencing their learning within the group.**

Supervision: Supervision provides the facilitator with the opportunity to: relate progress in academic learning, to the setting of different goals as appropriate, to the involvement of students directly in planning and evaluating their learning experiences, and to relating each of these elements to other phases and aspects of their overall development. For example, a student who is beginning to separate and accept the range of feelings he experiences and now needs to spend time in trying to evaluate the actual source of those feelings. Moreover, the on-going supervision of practising helpers is widely recognised as both desirable and essential for both their practise, and personal development, as practitioners. Supervision assists the helper in developing their own **internal supervisor** that they can have access to while they are working, and enable them to identify issues which they may then choose to bring to their formal supervision. For example:

☐ What was I hearing the client say and/or seeing the client do?

☐ What was I thinking and feeling about my observations?

☐ What were my alternatives to say and do at that point?

☐ How did I choose from among the alternatives?

☐ How did I intend to proceed with my selected response/s?

☐ What did I actually do/achieve with my response?

☐ What effect did my response have on the client? and

☐ How, then, might I evaluate the effectiveness of my response?

It is worth reminding ourselves that there are four beliefs that get in the way of adults learning:

☐ I must be competent

☐ I must be in control

☐ I must be consistent, and

☐ I must be comfortable

The belief that we have to be 'super-competent', is the problem, as opposed to being someone who remains open, needing to learn, wishing to learn, and also open about our vulnerabilities.

<u>Personal learning and group experience:</u> this is directly related to student progress within the actual experiential group environment where new learning is being applied, which is the very essence of training and development. The facilitator will have the benefit of having observed a student 'in practice' within the group. He will be monitoring and evaluating with the learner the feelings, attitudes, appreciations, values, and ideals, as they 'surface', develop, and change, during the training processes.

The above features must be an integral part of the learning process. **Self-evaluation, and the monitoring of personal progress is critically important for the student (and patient) to be aware of, and that activity, and responsibility, is also part of being a good practitioner.**

What is an Experiential Learning Group Like?

Inherent within an experiential learning group is what may be called, its therapeutic aspect. An appropriately convened experiential group is not without structure. The physical structure is achieved by all students sitting in a circle. The psychological structure is achieved initially by the facilitator providing a sense of security, safety, and nurture to the group. Members of the group normally speak one at a time. This, in turn, influences and structures behaviour within the group. Helping others in the group equals the sharing of their experience. **The essential principle is that students have the opportunity to think for themselves, explore attitudes, feelings, and judgements, which may then become the subject matter for the group.**

The climate of discussion in the group is informal, and is as permissive as possible, so that group members will feel free to say what they like. Of course, the freedom to speak does not come easily to some of us, in fact, some people will not speak freely about things that really matter to them until they feel they can trust the group with what they have to say. Essentially, helping equals the sharing of experience, therefore learning and personal development will be constrained unless we attempt to share our experience/s.

No one will share their experience until they are 'ready' to do so, and the depth of disclosure will also depend on a 'readiness to do so' as well as the degree of trust present.

When an experiential learning group is working to capacity students gain insight into the nature of behaviour, and personal growth, by the study of their experience rather than relying entirely upon formal instruction. Students are expected to learn from what happens in the group and from the facilitator's interventions. Such interventions must be about reinforcing learning through sensitive support, and enabling comment, rather than an authoritarian style or attitude.

As might be expected the first problem with the group is the problem of participation. The facilitator has to guide and provide a conceptual framework regarding group processes and particular aspects of group functioning if participation is to be achieved for all. Such guidance rests upon feedback. The principle function of the facilitator within the learning process is to help clarify, give meaning, and 'interpret'....that is, giving **feedback** as to what is happening in the group.

Giving and receiving feedback: such feedback will include:

- identifying the possibility of subgroups forming

- drawing out particularly significant teaching points

- detecting and commenting upon resistance to learning

- 'non-involvement' of some individuals by way of silence or withdrawal

- and of course, providing direction

The facilitator will attempt to ensure that fear of feedback is absent by maintaining trust, sense of security, and openness so that students will in fact participate in, and engage in, continuing and meaningful self-disclosure, and authenticity.

Giving, and receiving feedback, is often fraught with difficulty. The feelings surrounding feedback often lead to the feedback being badly given, in doing so, the fear of giving and receiving feedback is often reinforced. Feedback is essential to developing the learner's competence and confidence, at all stages in their development, with the most effective feedback being that based upon observable behaviours, case-based discussions, and so on. By incorporating feedback within learning, which emphasises reflective practice, helps learners to develop their own capacity for self-evaluation. Feedback should also be aligned with the overall learning outcomes of the given programme, or process.

It is essential to be **clear** about what the feedback is that you wish to give. Being vague and faltering will increase the anxiety in the receiver, and as such may obstruct understanding, ownership, learning, and participation in the process. Remember, the feedback you give is your own perception and not an ultimate truth! Therefore, feedback may say as much about the giver as it does about the receiver. It will help matters if within the feedback, phrases like, for example, 'I find you...' rather than 'You are...' are used. Try to give feedback as close to the event as possible, and balance negative and positive feedback. Be specific, as generalised feedback is hard to learn from. When giving feedback it is also important to make recommendations for change, and always to be constructive. Having a good professional relationship with learners will naturally help feedback to be received more appropriately.

Learning occurs through involvement in the experience itself as well as in any discussion that follows. Specific skills are improved through trial and error, feedback from others, the separation of feelings from behaviour, and 'old' thinking patterns. This can only be achieved through increased self-awareness and insight, and in the confidence of being able to express feelings openly and in an acceptable way. **The essence of gaining 'insight' is to be able to feel, and think about what you feel, at the same time you are feeling.**

Setbacks, Issues, and Problems:

Many students involved in the training to be helpers, and clients seeking help, may be experiencing a period of life transition for themselves. Many learners may already have completed one career be it as a parent, or other workplace setting. Not only will students and helpees bring differences in experience and differences in abilities, they will also bring preferred learning patterns, for example, self-directive learning versus a formal lecture structure.

Particular students may fail to see the purpose of either the conceptual input or the experiential exercises. They may also fail to see the links between the two. Teaching abstract concepts, for example, theories associated with cognitive development, may be seen by some as more advanced and superior to the use of more concrete methods of learning. All methods of teaching have their strengths and weaknesses, and their appropriate place.

The facilitator must recognise individual learning differences, that is, if students are to shift from being mere 'observers' in a learning process to being directly involved in the learning experience. Learning, from being directly involved in a given experience (including the experience of effective treatment), progresses as follows:

☐ engaging with the experience

☐ reviewing the experience

☐ drawing conclusions from the experience; and

☐ planning subsequent steps on the basis of that experience

Moreover, it is likely, especially at the start of a training course, that students may resent the 'group-therapy' aspect of the training because they perceive themselves as not necessarily requiring such. Other learners may fear that self-disclosure will involve the opening of a Pandora's Box. Remember, **people only reveal what they are ready to reveal**.

In accepting one of the core principles of helping, that is, the ability to put helpees at ease, the facilitator or helper has direct responsibility for putting their respective student or patient at ease. Direct experience is the best teacher, and group learning provides an ideal means of providing learners with the opportunity to gain direct experience in helping, and of personal growth and development.

The best facilitator has not directing from the outside, or from above, but is part of the group. He is, of course, seen by the group as a facilitator with special skills and experience and therefore different from the other group members. He is essential to the learning of the group which cannot, in fact, do without him. The facilitator is able to perform his role in the way that he does because he has already learned what the group is trying to learn. He can feel and observe and think at the same time. He can be emotionally involved, and know to what extent he is involved, and must be able to handle any transfer of feelings onto him whilst showing the others how to handle those feelings.

Furthermore, the facilitator must enable the group to understand the functions of authority, and this is likely to be expressed in his ability to accept, from the group, hostility, and thus show the group how to handle hostility. Nevertheless, there will always be setbacks especially when people feel that they are learning nothing and wasting their time. It has to become the material of the group, as will open disagreement, and interpersonal conflict.

Central to experimental learning is 'here and now' work. In other words, using what is actually happening in the here and now in the group as the material for discussion, analysis, feedback, learning, and then relating same to the helping process, and the helping of self and others.

What cannot be discounted is that the group meets with the knowledge that its members are there to work and the members would be quite opposed to the idea of doing nothing. It is also difficult for individuals within the group to do nothing as there is a need for individuals to be in contact with the 'emotional life' of the group. The dynamics of this appear to be: the relationship between the emotional state of the group, and that part of a given individual's need to participate and be involved in the group.

It would be counterproductive to achieving the overall aims of the training session to restrict the group, in such a way, that only pleasant emotions were experienced by members. Change involves discomfort. Yet, if the degree of discomfort is excessive then change will not take place and it is reasonably predictable that regressive behaviours and attitudes will then be pursued.

'.....the stimulus, the power, the motive of personal growth, these only come from the person himself and it can so easily be blocked and frustrated when it could be encouraged and developed.....'
(Rogers C R, 1982.)

Needless to say, the simplest way in estimating progress of the group (or therapeutic practice!) is the rate of dropout and attendance record. Obviously, a reasonable facilitator would be most concerned if things appeared to be going wrong. The preservation of the group may need to take precedence over any group activity.

There are two sets of influences which can threaten the existence of the group:

☐   disruptive forces from without, for example, poor administration of the course, and

☐   disorganising forces from within, for example persistent power struggles within the group

The facilitator must be on the watch for disintegration otherwise the group would become ineffective, decay, or break-up. (Berne E, 1983.) Nevertheless, it must be equally borne in mind that students join groups and maintain attendance, to a large extent, because they like being with the other members. They will be with people with whom they share certain interests, attitudes, and experiences, which contain their own value, and they are, of course, motivated toward helping, and gaining new insights.

The facilitator will be constantly monitoring the 'health' of the group, its etiquette, and progress. The problems involved in the survival of a group are as well illustrated in small groups as in nations. The facilitator endeavours to ensure the orderly survival of the group, and in doing so, in conjunction with group members, is keen to establish a rewarding and meaningful environment.

Resistance to change and new experiences has been acknowledged earlier. W R Bion (1961) in his seminal work 'Experiences in Groups and Other Papers' draws a similar parallel of the individual, the small group, and nations as follows:

'.... the neurotic patient does not want treatment, when at last his distress drives him to it he does not want it wholeheartedly.... society is not yet driven to seek treatment of its psychological disorders by psychological means because it has not achieved sufficient insight to appreciate the nature of its distress... the organisation of the training wing had to be such that the growth and insight should at least not be hindered....'

The helper's task then is to capitalise on the many motives already present in sufficient abundance within any learner and to harness these towards the attainment of the stated objectives. When the student acknowledges the real purpose and benefits of group work (or individual work) there will be no problem in maintaining participation for he will work with enthusiasm, initiative, and perseverance. Involvement will result in greater effort, greater understanding, greater enjoyment, and under these circumstances learning becomes real indeed.

CHAPTER THREE

Exploring Our Inner World

In developing the training and therapeutic model for helpers, the selection of the core material must be influenced by the principle of choosing the sequence of experiences aimed at promoting the student's maximum self-realisation rather than teaching a particular subject. It is the experiences incorporated into, and provided by the learning material, through which desirable learning takes place.

In one sense the subject matter is incidental to learning and is worthwhile only to the extent to which it enables the student to do something which is purposeful and growth enhancing. A basic tenet of non-directive counselling is that, as the individual perceives himself and situations differently, his behaviour will change accordingly. This clearly implies an attitude change particularly as attitudes underlie behaviour in such a fundamental way that it is necessary for students to **understand attitudes if they are to understand behaviour – especially as attitudes tend to become generalised into an overall outlook permeating all aspects of an individual's life.**

Attitudes:

Each of us has positive and negative feelings about many things. These positive and negative feelings about factors within our psychological world are our attitudes. Milton Rosenberg (1960) argued that people hold positive attitudes towards anything that helps them to obtain goals, and negative attitudes towards whatever blocks goal attainment. An attitude thus may be seen as a blend of belief and value – a feeling about a particular object in terms of its assumed relationship to one's values.

In Plato's terminology, attitudes combine cognitive (belief) and effective (value) components, few scientists assume that any specific attitudes are inborn. Carl Jung (1934), proposed the existence of inborn archetypes – unconscious predispositions towards certain patterns of thought and behaviour – upon which conscious attitudes may be based. However, his evidence was scientifically questionable. Hans Eysenck (1954) hypothesised that inherited differences in how particular individuals respond to external influences leads to a 'tough minded/tender minded' personality dimension which, in turn, predisposed people to adopt certain kinds of attitudes. Nevertheless, whatever their source, the development of attitudes is probably best explained through a multiple approach.

Attitudes may be the outcome of imitation of significant persons, for example, family or friends. They may also occur as a result of deliberate teaching, and as by-products of an emotional experience. The effective helper will realise attitudes are an important aspect of the self-concept as attitudes affect feeling, thinking and behaviour. Once developed, attitudes like values, tend to resist change especially when they are part of the anchor system of an individual's personality structure.

Therefore, attitudes may be thought of as learned patterns or behaviour which predisposes an individual to act in a specific way towards certain persons, objects or ideas. Gordon Allport (1935) defined an attitude as:

'...a state of readiness organised through experience exerting a directive and/or dynamic influence on the individual's response toward all objects or situations with which it is related....'

To the extent of an individual's current attitude serving a need, the individual is not likely to want to discard them, unless he is assured that the new attitudes provide greater satisfaction. Change of attitude, it must be remembered, like any other learning, is dependent upon motivation.

A person whose attitude toward the consumption of alcohol involves him in drinking six pints of beer a day will continue to do so until a change in attitude follows. Furthermore, he must be given the opportunity to experience satisfaction in connection with any new attitudes they will be reinforced by new behaviours. In other words, he will not revise his drinking habits until there is an adequate degree of motivation and reward present.

The thinking, feeling and behaving components associated with attitudes will exist at various levels of intensity and in various degrees of independence from one another. **Attitudes permeate our very existence.** The **self-concept,** for example, is best viewed as a complex system of attitudes and values which the individual has developed concerning himself in relation to his internal and external world. Consequently, attitudes arise as the by-products of one's day-to-day experiences and, therefore: **everything that goes on in the helping relationship as it affects the helpee (or student) leads to the formation or revision of attitudes.**

As already suggested, attitudes and values have no independent existence outside human thought and feeling – attitudes are heavily influenced by values and values are dependent in part on attitudes.

Yet, despite their resistance to change, attitudes are constantly being modified. Although change in attitude occurs more readily and more smoothly in people open to experience, every individual is constantly being forced to reappraise his attitudes as he interacts with his environment.

Given that attitudes are so basic to an individual's self-structure, a direct attack often only serves to intensify and solidify his attitudes as he endeavours to maintain a self-consistency. A gradual approach slowly brings about more permanent changes in attitudes than does an over assertive confrontation. It is necessary for such work to be undertaken in a permissive atmosphere in which the student (or the helpee) can express his attitudes without fear of threat or fear.

The more insecure the student or helpee the more likely he is to hold on to negative attitudes. Therefore it follows that the helper will do well to first consider how given attitudes support and are part of his self-concept. The use of an **attitude checklist** is extremely helpful in supporting people to give a more objective evaluation and concrete exposure to their attitudes, enabling them to reflect upon their attitudes, their desirability, and continuing relevance to their evolving self-concept.

There are numerous attitude checklists on the market, designed for different purposes, and measuring attitudes within different situations and circumstances. For example, the 'Revised Session Reactions Scale' (Elliot R, 1993) evaluates the client's response to a therapy session. Other attitude checklists can be more general and used to stimulate discussion, personal work, exploring our emotional and thinking responses to the external world, how we identify and differentiate ourselves from other people. Exploring attitudes may include examining attitude statements like:

☐   I despise authority

☐   I support de-regulation of financial markets

☐   I believe Marxist economics are relevant today

☐   I think it's a women's right to decide about abortion

☐   Sixteen-year old people should be allowed to drive cars

☐   I believe capital punishment is a correct deterrent

☐   In my opinion, film is the best form of entertainment

☐   Women are the stronger sex, and

☐   Education creates equality

Students will be asked to verbalise and generalise their attitudes in order to test and/or extend the scope of their desirability. Our attitudes, (like values) help guide behaviour. Attitudes are largely cognitive concerning thought or 'knowledge', or what the individual may assume to be 'knowledge', rather than affective aspects of the self, concerning our emotions.

To the extent that helpers are often used as role models in influencing attitudes in helpees makes it an imperative that helpers' attitudes meet definite standards of suitability from the all important standpoint of exemplifying the requirement to promote self-government, self-worth, and the worth of others.

Hence, work on attitudes is very necessary. A valuable exercise in gaining insight is that of developing a list of our own attitudes. **(See Handout Two: List of Attitudes for Discussion and Development of Own List)**.

Values:

Values, like a belief, differ from attitudes in that they tend to be more generalised. Values are related to more broad goals residing within the individual whereas attitudes have more specific reference. Thus, tolerance toward a noisy neighbour is an attitude whereas 'tolerance' as an abstraction is a value.

Use of the term 'values', it is suggested, refers specifically to an individual's concept to **what is desirable**. When, for example, we identify a person's values as including 'happiness', 'security' and 'a loving family', we need not travel around the world seeking to discover an object called 'happiness' in order to demonstrate that we have located such a value.

NOTE: An attitude does not necessarily imply that a person will feel a need to behave in a certain way, whereas, a value tends to involve certain behaviours being defined as desirable.

In other words, a value does not specify one pattern of learned behaviour, nor does it have to specify a particular object of desire.

An attitude like 'I enjoy walking' is specific, whereas a value like 'people should respect others' has more subjective quality.

Individual values can range from the very general, the most abstract philosophical or religious concepts, to the highly specific and mundane. Values tend to stress concepts of ultimately desirable goals such as 'the greatest good for the greatest number' but, of course, an individual may possess no such concepts of ultimate states and focus instead on being able to 'feed myself when I am hungry'. Moreover, behaviour is affected by a hierarchy of values within the individual's self-concept.

Helping involves the helper in a clarification of values, how values might be changed, or incorporated into a meaningful self-concept, which is capable then of generating consistent growth-enhancing conduct.

If helping is to be successful in this area then it is necessary to have facilitators who themselves have fairly well-defined values which they display and express in consistent and meaningful ways so that students can see that values are something one lives by, rather than something one just talks about.

Effecting values and altering attitudes is part of the helping process. This will be discussed further in the section on problem solving, particularly as values and attitudes themselves are of tremendous importance to the private and social life of every individual and, regardless of how they might be defined, are held by all of us.

In essence, attitudes and values transform our personal world view from a small set of animal perceptions to the vast array of ideas and views that will embrace unequal parts of certainty and mystery, good and evil, enthusiasm and disinterest. Values and attitudes are psychological constructs, that is, they cannot be observed directly by another individual but are inferred through what an individual might say, and how he behaves.

Each of us is the organisation of values and attitudes into a single system that constitutes our 'self concepts'. It is very useful indeed for understanding the things we actually value by objectively developing a list of values we can own for ourselves. **(See Handout Three, (and Handout Seven): A Values List for Discussion and Development of Own List).**

Self-concept:

Building the self-concept involves a slow process of selection and rejection of attitudes and values, the selection and rejection of a range of influences, from which gradually emerges a sense of awareness which defines more clearly just who and what we are. A T Jersild, (1952) provides the following definition:

'....a person's self is the sum total of all that he can call his. The self includes, among other things, a certain system of ideas, attitudes, values, and commitments. The self is a person's total subjective environment; it is the distinctive centre of experience and significance. The self constitutes a person's inner world as distinguished from the outer world consisting of all other people and things.....'

The self-concept, therefore, has crucial implications for our development as an individual. **Our self-concept stands at the centre of what we do or do not do in our attempt to maintain a unified self.**

A self-concept will draw upon, in addition to values and attitudes, a range of reference points, for example, physique, intelligence, musical talent, being a mother, being a man, and so on. The adequacy of the self-concept which we develop out of our interactions with the environment is indeed the result of incredibly complex processes, and these are ongoing.

Our self-concept has crucial implications for our development and as such can be attested within the helping environment where day after day, helpers are working with people who are involved in a desperate attempt to maintain a unified self and in doing so often cling onto destructive and short-sighted modes of behaviour.

The pattern of life of every individual is a living out of his or her self-image. Hence, **when we resist learning**, which might otherwise be beneficial to us, it is likely that **we are trying to safeguard a picture of ourselves.** This self picture may be forced and unhealthy but it is the only one we know.

It is only under conditions of security that we can afford to release the barriers and explore new options. Our defences certainly keep things out, but they also keep things in! Our defences may indeed 'protect us' because, for example, we cannot tolerate failure, or admit inadequacy, but at the same time these defences prevent us from exploring new options in meeting our real potentialities.

Clearly, it is important for each of us to feel good about ourselves in order that we might grow and fulfil our full potential. A self-image associated with 'I am a failure' or for example, 'I will be a success at all costs' contains potentially destructive and counterproductive influences on any growth continuing.

Abraham Maslow (1960) is of major importance in any debate on the idea of self-concept. In introducing work on attitudes, values, and self-concept Maslow's **'Inventory of Self-actualizing Characteristics'** (ISAC) is an invaluable tool not only for work involving helpees but for all of us. Maslow's work has made a significant and lasting effect upon the entire field of psychology. I suggest no other study of healthy people (most psychodynamic studies have tended to focus on psychological sickness) even approaches his influence. His model of self-actualizing people has stood the test of time for almost 50 years, and has proven, to this day, to be a powerful idea about living life at its best which has yet to be matched in psychology to this day.

Moreover, the ISAC is an instrument which looks at personality traits as well as values and attitudes, and the exploration of *questions* associated with 'interpersonal style' and *statements* on 'interpersonal style' are more than worthy of utilisation. **(See Handout Four: Questions about my Interpersonal-Style, and Handout Five: Statements on my Interpersonal-Style)**

<u>**Maslow's Construct of the Self-actualizing Person**</u> is based upon his study of those characteristics that differentiated the 'most remarkable human beings' from ordinary persons. He reviewed the lives of many people, famous and unknown, living and dead, to discover the behaviours that led some human beings to a pattern of excellence in everyday living. His **belief in the human capacity to grow in quality shaped the human potential movement within the field of psychology.**

Before higher needs can become important or a priority for us we must first have our more basic needs met, such as food, safety, shelter, belonging. Then we are free to concentrate on the higher needs and values, enabling us to become self-actualizing, 'happy and productive'. Consider Maslow's list of characteristics of self-actualization as a role model and guide! **(See Handout Six: Maslow's Characteristics of Self-actualized People)**

Maslow never actually arrived at a **definition of self-actualization** as he viewed it as an ongoing process that involved:

'...full use and exploitation of talents, capacities, potentialities....as such people seem to be fulfilling themselves and to be doing the best that are capable of doing....'

Self-actualizing persons were seen by Maslow as being free of neurotic, psychopathic, or psychotic tendencies. Their basic needs for safety, belongingness, love, and self-respect were gratified. Self-actualization is not necessarily to be equated with fame or to achievement.

The genius of the self-actualizing person is poured into his or her everyday life.

Maslow's list of 'virtues' of the self-actualizing person described attitudes, behaviours, and characteristics of the person in the process of developing his full state.

'...self-actualizing persons are not saints. They have many of the 'lesser human failings'; however, the self-actualizing person is aware of his imperfections, owns them, and makes choices about keeping or overcoming the undesirable traits...'

The ISAC is based directly on Maslow's descriptions of the self-actualizing person. It is designed for two purposes to teach in some detail the concept of self-actualization, and to provide a people with a device for measuring their own self-actualizing process.

As a self feedback instrument, the ISAC can be used in any training situation in which a focus on self-appraisal, personal growth, or individual goal setting is desired. (Banet, A.G 1976)

The ISAC consists of 75 items, five derived from each of Maslow's 15 characteristics of self-actualising persons. Helpees often find this to be a useful instrument in clarifying where they might be on the continuum of self-actualization but also provides areas and topics for personal work.

The characteristics interrogated in the ISAC include 'acceptance of self, others, human nature', 'freshness of appreciation', 'un-hostile sense of humour', and 'capacity for peak experiences'. Not only does the inventory provide a vehicle for self-exploration, as suggested above, but also provides material which can later be used by the respective student, or within the group to enhance further self-exploration and understanding.

Students who score low, for example, in 'acceptance of self, others, human nature', will have the opportunity to examine that particular finding against their overall world view including attitudes, values, and self-concept.

The first step in growth or improvement of self, is to identify the incompatible parts of ourselves and then giving them up, or integrating them into a meaningful whole.

The issue is basically one concerning change or modification of one's self-concept. The answer lies in providing students (and of course helpees) with an atmosphere in which the individual can afford to reconsider, in safety, old as well as new perceptions, and to integrate them in a way which is meaningful. Within such an atmosphere individuals are free from having to cling to, in a defensive way, old attitudes, values, and behaviours.

Growth implies a gradual evolution through assimilation of new experiences, and self-discovery through new insights which then may be incorporated into a new and more adequate self-image.

Growth involves the rejection of incompatible ideas and the adoption of new attitudes and values which gradually erode incompatible behaviours. Like the ISAC, a 'Trait Checklist' provides an additional vehicle for students of helping and helpees to examine for themselves, and later explore within the group, particular traits which they may wish to give up, and others which they may with to develop. **(See Handout Eight: A Trait Checklist)**

Numerous checklists, standardised tests, and personality measures are available. They will differ in validity and specific benefit. Their use is basically a matter of choosing the most appropriate instrument in terms of a specific purpose, related to the given training, or therapeutic goal. They can provide information from which further work can be planned. The use of checklists directly invite self-report and feedback. They also avoid 'measurement' of performance.

Students can be invited to work on, for example, a trait checklist which involves not only examining a prepared list of possible traits but also provides the opportunity for self-evaluation. Trait checklists vary in length and are based upon the attitudes one may hold towards oneself and, by implication, affects not only one's own behaviour but how one views others. For example, a prepared checklist of traits may include statements similar to:

☐ I like myself

☐ I say wrong things

☐ I do not enjoy being the sex I am

☐ I believe life has little meaning

☐ I have trouble controlling my feelings

☐ I use my talents, and

☐ I believe much of my life is a charade, etc.

Moreover, as with Maslow's 'Inventory of Self-actualizing Characteristics' which serves our search regard to enhancing self-awareness, a trait checklist can be utilised along with, for example, statements on values, in achieving a similar purpose.

As we discussed above, a values checklist provides a list of statements which invites us to accept them (or reject them) as our own. Values accepted are, of course, as important in understanding oneself as the ones which are rejected. The examples below suggest how work on the two lists together will have the potential to be extremely productive.

- ☐ I believe: it important to help the sick and needy

- ☐ to be in complete harmony with the universe

- ☐ to rid the world of injustice

- ☐ it is important to be with the family

- ☐ to be the richest person in the world

- ☐ to protect the environment, etc.

In examining material arising from the use of checklists it is possible to explore with the students not only the notion or their own self-concept but also their own **self-ideal.** This is extremely useful as it begins to identify the level of expectation an individual sets for himself, and thus determines the kind of self-concept he is likely to develop.

The need for a realistic level of aspiration follows directly from the need for the self-concept to maintain contact with reality. What an individual achieves or fails to achieve is meaningful only with reference to the target towards which the individual was, or is, aiming.

An issue worthy of consideration here is the inability of the 'unaware person' to set realistic goals. The 'unaware person' finds it difficult to tolerate failure or to admit his lack of 'awareness'. He often sets for himself impossible goals which he attempts desperately to attain, or which he uses as an excuse for his inadequacy. The more self-aware individual sets goals for himself in keeping with his potential, and is content to accept a measured improvement in his performance and achievement of goals.

The fact that helping operates on an interpersonal dimension means that the personal development of socially adequate behaviour is essential for the helper. Socially adequate behaviour is primarily a matter of developing a self-concept in which one's needs and purposes are integrated with those of the helpee, that is, they are goal-directed, and therefore contains mutual benefit for both.

One's emotions, of course, play a part. Our emotions are such an integral part of our total personality and are important because of the way in which they motivate behaviours and, therefore, influence our social interaction. The helping relationship and experiential learning environment provide exactly such a real opportunity, and setting, to explore emotions and feelings.

Emotions and Feelings:

As noted above, emotions and feelings are an integral part of the total personality and, therefore, are of critical concern in helping. A broad range of conditions and circumstances arouse emotion and equally a broad range of emotions are 'stirred up', and they will equally vary in intensity.

Emotions affect the body, for example increased heartbeat, and range from conditions such as joy to sadness, and from irritation to satisfaction. In our workplace and no doubt in our homes, we encounter temper, jealousy, despondency, as well as laughter. The range of emotional behaviour for which each of us is capable is considerable and is likely to vary from person to person. Some people have 'preferred' feelings, for example, 'feeling depressed' as a learned response to life, and as such, individuals learn to define themselves in this way. The more self-aware person leads a richer emotional life and understands and appreciates his emotions for what they are, and utilises and integrates them for his own welfare, and that of others. He is not emotionless, but as a result of his personal stability, channels his emotions and the energy from which he generates constructive behaviours.

The feeling associated with an emotion is the most important part of the emotion – it may even be considered to be the emotion!

For example, 'feelings' described as irritation, jealousy, ambivalence, incompetence, amazement, are emotional states which involve feelings. It is absolutely essential in helping to ensure that when someone is describing an emotion the actual feeling behind the emotion is qualified. For a person to say 'I feel inadequate' is not enough, and is not the sharing of a feeling. The feeling behind 'inadequacy' might be fear, anger, or sadness. **It is impossible to work effectively in helping unless the root feeling behind an emotional state is confirmed.** Once confirmed the helper will then know exactly which feeling response he is dealing with. The helper could introduce work which encourages 'confidence' in place of 'inadequacy' without taking account of, for example, the (un-clarified) 'sadness' that was behind the patient's statement of 'inadequacy'.

In searching for the root feeling, or mixture of feelings, the helper will be searching from the helpee one of four feelings which lay behind all emotion. These are either (or a combination of, people may fear, and have anger and fear about the same issue):

- **fear**
- **anger**
- **sadness, and**
- **joy**

The aim here is to integrate the experience of 'feeling' into a coherent and personally satisfying learning and growing process. Before coherent learning and growing can happen it is necessary for people to:

- acknowledge the range of feeling/s or emotions they experience

- be aware of which feelings is actually being experienced

- why it is being experienced

- allow the experience

- be responsible for the experience, and

- and behave in ways, and make decisions, about the experience, that are ultimately self-enhancing

54

Thinking and Feeling:

Many people are often 'lazy' about thinking, or have not had appropriate experience in the use of their ability to think. Part of the helping process is about encouraging people to provide genuine self-disclosure. It is also about eliciting from them, from what they bring, issues from their own thinking. It is also about encouraging people to ask the same questions of themselves without resorting to 'maladaptive' responses or modes of interacting, in other words, encouraging genuine self-disclosure by enabling the helpee to progressively **think with clarity.**

Thinking is often confused with feeling. As suggested in the previous section there are four feelings expressive of emotion. What is also true is that people often offer a thought, when asked for a feeling. This confusion must be encountered by repeating the request for a feeling. In this way, people begin to distinguish their thoughts and their feelings, and become more congruent in their responses. For example:

Helper: 'How do you feel about being here now?'

Helpee: 'We are going to tea in a minute'

Helper: 'What are you feeling about being here now?'

Helpee: 'Nothing'

Helper: 'That's what you are thinking. What are you feeling?'

Helpee: 'Sad'

One of the main goals of helping is to help the person deal in straight and genuine ways, with his feelings, wants, and needs as they occur.

The helpee must be given permission to express his feelings appropriately instead of just accepting 'I don't feel', and must be given permission to think instead of using replies which say 'I can't think'.

The capacity to think, and to think about feelings, must be expected of everyone no matter what the level of their problem or 'disturbance' might be. Confronting confusions between thinking and feeling is in itself therapeutic, as it begins to re-order an otherwise 'chaotic' internal world. Moreover, by encouraging the open expression of thought, and ownership of feelings, other agendas which the helpee may be aware of can be responded to, for example, a person may have learned that is not appropriate to express anger in an open way and consequently may have learned to deflect his anger as sarcasm, or cynicism.

Individuals must be held accountable for all their thoughts and feelings within the student group, or the therapeutic process, which arise from within themselves or occur as the result of transactions with others.

Each individual is responsible for checking what he thinks is occurring in him, or in his environment. Behaviours which seem inappropriate need to be challenged or confronted from a caring position. **Confrontation is equal to caring and doing nothing is equal to not caring.** In fact all interactions and interpersonal exchanges are expected to arise from the caring for oneself, and for the other person with whom the transaction is held. Mutual responsibility is a key factor in helping. Acting-out is no excuse for not knowing what to do or say in a particular situation. The expectation is that:

☐ the helpee will function in a coherent and responsible manner

☐ that he will take responsibility for what he needs to know, and

☐ for what he needs to do

Helping is about raising and bringing into the awareness of the helpee, the difficulties he may be experiencing, and exploring possible solutions to these difficulties through the dialectic relationship with the helpee.

Helping is an interpersonal event and therefore in order to further understand a student's motives in wishing to be a helper, and also to facilitate growth, the interpersonal dimensions of a student's life are worthy of examination. Such will include addressing questions like:

☐　　Do I wish to spend at lot of time with people?

☐　　Do I choose being with people who do what I wish?

☐　　Do I spend time with whoever comes along?

☐　　Do others know I care for them?

☐　　Which emotions do I enjoy with others?

☐　　Which emotions do I fear?

☐　　Am I easily hurt?

☐　　What do I do when I get hurt?

☐　　Do I see myself as selfish?

Again, the focus is providing the opportunity for the student to gain insight. Interpersonal behaviour does not just occur, but arises in response to some form of need. Human beings are besieged at all times with a range of needs, and only a few of these needs can be satisfied at any on time. Needs underlie every phase of human relations, and only when a helper is fully aware of this fact can he begin to provide effective help to others. **(See Handouts Four, Five, and Eight)**

Asking questions and exploring the answers related to our interpersonal behaviour is the beginning of understanding, moreover, by providing students with a range of statements concerning interpersonal style addresses the same issue and exposes the range of emotions that determine specific behaviours, for example:

☐　　I am a loving person

☐   I find it hard to face others

☐   I am self-controlled

☐   I am very easily hurt

☐   I am an anxious person

☐   I am impulsive

☐   I think others do not like me

☐   I have the courage of my convictions

☐   I do not let my emotions show

All of the foregoing material is orientated toward the learner who is to do the learning. Although essential to helping situations, this material is also focused toward the development of the helper in becoming a more self-aware person. What we think of ourselves revolves round our attitudes and values, and as such determine for us 'what is right and what is wrong' and 'what is adequate and inadequate'. Our continuous professional development, is indeed continuous, that is if we wish to continue referring to ourselves as being professional.

The exercises involve all of us in our own 'problem solving' and will confront them with varying degrees of discomfort. The key to effective educational experience, as in problem solving itself, relies to a large extent on individual motivation.

The student and the helpee will exert themselves with whatever capacity they can muster when they are working towards goals which are real and meaningful in terms of their motives and qualities. Lack of commitment can of course, negate the best efforts of all concerned. By providing a secure and safe learning environment the facilitator will stimulate motivation and encourage rather than impede learning, and self-discovery.

CHAPTER FOUR

<u>**Considering a Practical Theoretical Framework**</u>

Anyone who has worked in helping for a number of years will be impressed by a person's capacity to change, and also their resistance to change. This is not to say that people intentionally refuse to alter their behaviour or resolve personal difficulties, on the contrary, they are often the first to say 'I'm unhappy, I want to change'. It seems also to be true to say that many people have been so seriously affected by particular experiences or circumstances that they are impelled to remain unchanged, and cling to their established and habitual patterns of behaviour.

It would seem that many helpees are not in touch with what they want, other than to get rid of their pain, their confusion, their insecurity, and often these will be denied, denied because change is threatening, difficult, and uncertain. **Change only becomes possible for people if they know where they are, or have been, or know who they are and where they may wish to go.**

Transactional Analysis (TA) provides a theoretical response to such issues, and a therapeutic means of re-establishing appropriate communication in place of acting-out, and maladapted behaviour.

The thinking and feeling disorders behind many of the problems presented in the helping relationship are extremely complex to unravel. Most of us wish to change some aspects of our personality or life. **The nature of helping stresses the concept of personal growth, becoming more genuine, changing attitudes about ourselves, others, and the world.**

One of the difficulties of 'analysing' and so improving everyday behaviour with other people is that for the layman, the theories and writings of psychologists and social behaviourists have been very difficult to follow, because of both the language used, and the complexity of the conceptual ideas.

An extremely useful technique for fostering awareness and self-responsibility is TA. It is a systematic and methodical approach to human behaviour developed by Eric Berne in the early 1960s. It includes a way to answer those difficult questions about ourselves and our lives, such as:

☐ What is going on?

☐ Why is it going on?

☐ Why do I feel the way I do?

☐ I don't like what is going on?

☐ What can I do about it?

The language of TA is simple, its concepts are based on commonsense everyday observation of what we see and what we feel. Moreover, a useful level of understanding which can be put to practical use is available very quickly.

Essentially TA is a teaching and learning device rather than a confessional or an exploration of our psychic cellars. TA operates from the belief that we all have a natural tendency to live, to take care of ourselves, to be healthy. If we are unhealthy, unhappy, are uninterested in learning, it is the result of external or internal oppressive influences which overpower this inherent positive life tendency. Even when overpowered, this positive tendency remains dominant so that it is always ready to express itself when oppression lifts.

Each of us learns specific behaviours when growing up, and although our childhood decisions are strongly influenced by our parents and others, we in turn make decisions about ourselves and for ourselves. As we grow we begin to make and decide upon a life plan for ourselves and, therefore, by implication can change our life plan by making new decisions at any time. **Thus, we are responsible for our own growth as we alone exercise the choice to retain our old decisions or make new ones.**

No-one can make us change. Each of us is ultimately responsible only for himself and not for others.

Four Main Concepts:

TA encompasses four main concepts. The focus of these concepts is upon what is happening to the person 'Now'. A summary of each of the four main concepts is provided, followed by an explanation of some of the implications of the concepts within the change process. It is emphasised that the following is a brief overview particularly as numerous books on TA are available, in particular 'Games People Play' by Eric Berne (1964).

1.   Structural Analysis

This is the analysis of individual personality. It is a method of analysing a person's thoughts, feelings, and behaviours based on the phenomena of ego states. (It is important to understand that these ego states are not abstract concepts such as Sigmund Freud's concepts of ego, super ego, and id, but are states that can be observed.) Three ego states have been identified and their characteristics observed, evaluated, and carefully described. They are the Parent ego state, Child ego state, and the Adult ego state.

The **Parent ego state** is a collection of attitudes, thoughts and corresponding behaviours, incorporated from external sources, primarily parents or other significant adults. Outwardly, this ego state shows either critical or nurturing behaviour. It is concerned with helping, criticising, censoring, laying down rules, punishing, plus caring, forgiving, being permissive – in fact 'all the behaviour' we commonly associate with being a parent. Words and phrases which help identify when a person is in the Parent ego state would be: 'should', 'don't', 'ought', 'never', 'because I said so', 'are you comfortable?'.

We can begin to get in touch with our Parent ego state by becoming more aware of our actual parents, for example:

- How did they talk about money?

- Who could be relied upon?

☐ Did they have fun together?

☐ What were the maleness and femaleness messages?

☐ Who controlled the purse strings?

☐ How/what were household chores decided upon?

☐ Was their clothing clean and attractive?

☐ What did they say about education?

☐ What were the ethical, and moral values your, parents taught you?

☐ Did they express anger, or hate, or love towards you?

☐ Did they manipulate you? With guilt, fear, criticism, sweetness, false compliments?

☐ What mottoes or sayings were you reared on? Were these helpful, hurtful, or irrelevant?

☐ Do you think they encouraged you to be a winner or a loser?

Recollect your parents, as if there is a 'parent tape' going around in your head. Ask yourself the question, 'how do I copy them?' What is my Critical Parent ego state like, and how do I use it with my family, friends, and work colleagues? What is my Nurturing Parent ego state like and how do I use it with family, friends and work colleagues?

Our thoughts and behaviours have their roots deep in our history. As a child we watched and listened to our parents/carers, and those around us. We incorporated countless messages about ourselves, others, and the wider world. Are these given parental tapes still relevant and active in our life, positively or negatively, as well as the adaptations we may have needed to make? Think about the kind of messages that we receive from our parents: 'whatever is worth doing is worth doing right', 'that's girls work', 'don't blow your own trumpet', 'you can't trust men', 'you will never succeed', 'people like us...', and so on.

Thus on the basis of his experiences the child acquires his convictions, makes his decisions, and takes his position. He has no way of really telling facts from delusions, and most everyday events are distorted. His adapted strategies of behaviour are devised in an attempt to provide answers and comfort in the face of what appears to him the only way to react to an often threatening world, a place where he lives in an essentially subordinate position, with adults who have much more power than him.

The **Child ego state** contains all the impulses that come naturally to an infant, such as joy, trust, love. It also contains the recordings of our early experiences, how we were responded to, and the subsequent view or position taken about ourselves and others. Being in your Child ego state does not mean you are childish or foolish; it means you are feeling or acting like the little boy or girl you once were: a fit of temper, rolling down the hillside, giggling, having fun, feeling nervous, scared, anxious, inferior. Words and phrases would be: 'can't', 'won't', 'I'm scared', 'nobody loves me', 'do it for me'. In TA the Child ego state is seen as **the source from which the best in human beings comes** and is therefore the source of renewal in life.

Listen to the hurts, longings, and happiness of your inner child. Imagine yourself back at home say as a toddler, at five years of age, 10, as an adolescent. Let the pictures emerge. Responses that come from the Child ego state are usually emotionally charged. Even though we are adults, we have a 'child' inside. Remember that when in our Child ego state we feel and act like the little person we once were, full of impulses, feelings, creativity, spontaneity, fun, laughter, anger, fear, anger, joy, love, expressiveness, affectionate, playfulness, selfish, standing up for our rights, and so on. Think about:

☐ how you act when under stress

☐ how you respond when the child in another person invites or provokes the child in you

☐   when someone becomes critical of you

☐   when you are at a party

☐   when you feel happy

☐   when you feel sad

☐   when you feel angry

☐   when you want something

☐   when you are criticised, and

☐   what does your inner child believe about itself?

When we act and feel as we did in childhood we are in our Child ego state. The natural child feels free and does what he wishes to do, the Child ego state is the foundation of our self-image.

The **Adult ego state** is not related to the person's age. It contains those behaviours concerned with collecting and processing facts and information, trying to get in touch with objective reality, with testing probability. It is sometimes referred to as the 'computer' in the personality and operates dispassionately. Words and phrases would be: 'how many?', 'why?', 'what is the time?'. It is important to avoid using any value judgement in using these definitions of ego states. The Adult is not better than the Child or Parent, only different.

Implications for Change

An awareness and understanding of ego states provides a solid foundation for change. It enables us to make connections between our own inner world and our current transactions with others. A transaction is defined by Berne as follows:

'...if two or more people encounter each other...sooner or later one of them will speak, or give some other indication of acknowledging the presence of the others. This is called a transactional stimulus.

Another person will then say or do something which is in some way related to the stimulus, and that is called the transactional response...'

So, an awareness of the ego states helps us to understand more fully how the things that have happened to us affect us now. **By 'tracking' our ego states, we 'track' ourselves.** Hence our behaviours and responses can be constantly and consistently diagnosed. As we become aware of using an ego state inappropriately, our own self-monitoring system will make adjustments which then encourage clear and precise thinking. A statement like 'I don't care about myself' also implies, 'I don't care about others'. The 'I don't care about myself' comes from a Child ego state adaption and reflects a life position of 'I'm not OK, and not only am I not OK, but neither are others'.

It is the realisation that our growth is constrained by **the power struggle going on between our ego states, between Child wishes, Parent beliefs, and the rational Adult that enables us to identify and re-think the illusions governing our present actions.**

2.   Transactional Analysis

TA (the specific analysis of actual transactions) explains:

- ☐   why some interpersonal transactions are effective
- ☐   why other transactions lead to misunderstanding and cut people off from each other, and
- ☐   why some transactions are open and straight and others closed and defensive or phoney and crooked

TA helps us to observe how we use our ego states and how the ego states of one person interacts with the ego states of another.

Transactions may be classified as complementary, crossed, or ulterior. A transaction can be defined as complementary when we receive a response which shows we have been understood.

A Complementary Transaction:

Helper: "What time is your next appointment" (from Adult ego-state, to Adult ego state of the helpee/other person)

Helpee: "It is six o'clock." (from Adult ego state, to Adult ego state)

The stimulus given received the response expected, and was therefore complementary).

A Crossed Transaction:

Crossed transactions happen when the initial stimulus is crossed by an unexpected response. That is, the reply is sent to an ego state other than from the one it was sent.

Helper: "How are you today?" (from Parent ego state)

Helpee: "Go away, leave me alone!" (from Child ego state, to Child ego state of the Helper)

Ulterior transactions:

These are more complex than complementary or crossed transactions. They differ in that they always involve more than two ego states at the same time. When an ulterior message is sent it is disguised under a socially acceptable cover. For example:

'You are looking well today (sent from Nurturing Parent ego-state)... considering' (sent from Critical Parent ego state). This message could be received by two ego states – to Adult or Child. To the Adult ego state, 'You are looking well today', and to the Child ego state 'considering', such a response leaves the recipient feeling confused and criticised, and leaves the sender feeling superior and powerful.

Analysing transactions is a specialized and rewarding area of study. Gestures, facial expressions, body posture, tone of voice, and so, all contribute to the meaning in every transaction. (Professionally recognised courses are available, and the

International Transactional Analysis Association is contactable at www.itaa-net.org).

Implications for change

It is important to identify the nature of our transactions. Are we sending confused and confusing messages, which quickly convey acceptance, caring, or rejection of others?

Which ego state do we use most often, which are avoided, how do we respond to messages from different ego states, do we cross transactions, do we use different ego states to transact with men or than with women? Answers to these questions can provide a great deal of useful information about how to maintain and enjoy open communication, about what each of our ego states is thinking, feeling or doing, and how to avoid transactions which are destructive to us.

3. **Game Analysis**

Games are transactions between people which are always destructive at least to one of the players. So why do we engage in them? Basically, because of our past experience of strokes, **a stroke is a stimulation one person gives to another; it may be positive or negative, a kiss or a cuff.** The legacy of experience leads us to seek the kind of situation where we are 'justified' in indulging in our favourite feelings or emotions – anger, martyrdom, failure, or whatever. Many psychological games have been identified. For example, 'Kick Me' players go around getting into trouble or doing things which invite punishment or criticism.

Such people feel life has always been against them and they look for confirmation of this by getting people to 'Kick' them. 'Wooden Leg' is a psychological game where people use some real or imaginary handicap as an excuse for not achieving anything… 'what do you expect of me, I suffer from hay fever?' It is like saying 'what can you expect of a poor person with a wooden leg?' Rather than going ahead and doing whatever is possible, the person plays the game. A person playing this game uses a handicap – social, physical, educational, personal background – in order to manipulate others.

People play games because people learn to believe certain things about themselves and others. When people play games people play act roles. **Victims** play to collect bad feelings but they also encourage others to feel angry, frustrated, or guilty. **Rescuers and Persecutors** play to give bad feelings, yet also collect arrogance, 'purity', superiority and hostility. 'I only count when people are paying attention to me – scolding, nagging, criticising', or 'I only count when I am rescuing others', for example, 'Don't you worry, I'll clear up the mess'.

Games played by Victims, Rescuers, and Persecutors include as follows:

Persecutors: (involve anger/triumph)

☐ Now I've got you
☐ If it weren't for you
☐ See what you made me do
☐ Why don't
☐ Look at the mess you made
☐ Blemish (finding fault)

Rescuers: (involve concern/pity)

☐ I'm only trying to help you
☐ What would you do without me
☐ They'd be glad they knew me
☐ Always happy to help

Victims: (grief/confusion)

☐ Wooden leg
☐ Kick Me
☐ Why does this always happen to me?
☐ I'm stupid
☐ Poor me
☐ Addict (alcoholic etc.)
☐ Harried

The payoff for playing games is the manipulation of others in order to experience favourite feelings. This form of self-indulgence is called **Rackets.**

Game players always find a 'partner' with whom to play. Games are played on what is called the drama triangle: the Rescuer rescues the Victim, then the actual victim persecutes the Rescuer, so the actual Rescuer is now the Victim, the once rescuer, now victim, will now persecute the new victim the person he originally wished to rescue...and around it goes. The helpful advice for everyone is, if you find yourself on the drama triangle, get off quick, and find some one with whom you are able to have genuine, rewarding, and 'straight' transactions!

Rackets relate to the drama triangle as follows:

The persecutor, 'I am better than you, you are inferior'. The game is, Blemish.

The victim, 'I am helpless you are better than me'. The game is, Kick Me.

The rescuer, 'I am okay (if) I help others, they are inadequate'. The game is, 'I am only trying to help you'.

Games can be played at three levels:

- first degree: a mild game which leaves people feeling mildly uncomfortable

- second degree: has quickly escalated into a serious argument, or where a game has gone on for a couple of days and has escalated into a situation where very powerful emotions are involved

- third degree: this level may involve tissue damage, hospital, jail, or morgue

A helpful way of identifying if you are playing psychological games, and the roles you may be playing within games, or if you are getting caught up in other people's games, is to consider the following questions:

☐ What keeps happening over and over again in particular relationships?

☐ How does it get started?

☐ What happens next?

☐ And then what happens?

☐ How does it end? and

☐ How do I feel after it ends?

The skilled helper will deal with Games in several ways, some of which include:

☐ bringing the game into the helpee's awareness

☐ confront the discounting that is involved, and

☐ and to encourage the helpee to ask for what it is they really want

Aware individuals can determine the course of their own life plans and rewrite these 'dramas' with their own uniqueness, avoid games, and the roles of victim, persecutor, or rescuer, and confront these roles, and script themes.

Implications for Change

Games provide many strokes and they are not easily given up. Once we identify the games we play we can gradually learn to function in more genuine ways. We can learn to attract fewer put-downs and to pass out better feelings, to be 'real' more of the time, rather than to act out roles, to do more things ourselves, risk sharing more of ourselves, to laugh at our games. Every time we take a positive step, to becoming more genuine, and by giving up 'play' behaviours, we begin to exchange warmer, more positive feelings, increase our chances not only of growing and realising more fully our potential, but also **better health.**

4.   **Script Analysis**

A script is a blueprint by which we live our lives. It is formed by all the messages that are mediated to the growing person from birth into adolescence. Many of these messages are simple **proscriptions or prescriptions** (to proscribe is to outlaw, to ostracize, to prohibit or denounce; to prescribe is to lay down a rule or direction, give an order, to set boundaries), and these messages further influence and help define to the growing child:

☐   what and who he is

☐   what he is to become, and

☐   what kind of chronicle of events he can expect to live through

Let us think about **how influences may have been internalized** by asking ourselves a few general questions:

☐   Did any one ever tell you what you would be good at, if so what, and are you doing it, or something similar?

☐   What messages did you receive about what was Ok or not Ok for you to do because of your gender?

☐   Who was the most important person in setting your life goals, how do you now think and feel about the outcome?

☐   What kind of strokes did you get, and how have these affected your script decisions?

☐   How was work looked at by your family?

☐   When you were in secondary school did any of your teachers think you had special talents, if so what? If no, do you believe early decisions and choices about your life were affected?

☐ Today, are you in any way living up to the expectations, negative or positive, of your teachers or significant others?

Some scripts are very destructive and are programming a person into a life of failure. Underlying messages may be 'get lost' or 'be stupid' or 'fail'. In daily life we experience or observe in ourselves and others, a compulsion to perform in a certain way, to live up to a specific identity, to fulfil a destiny. To the extent that script messages are not in tune with our actual potential, they negate our will to function effectively and therefore create disharmony. **We, in fact, become absurd caricatures of our possible selves.**

You probably know someone who is moving towards a tragic ending – suicide or its equivalent, such as alcoholism, drugs, or obesity. You probably know someone who is fighting to get to the top, no matter what the cost to self or others. You also probably know someone who keeps going around in circles, never getting anywhere, or merely existing instead of really living. **Our script will always be based on three questions which involve identify and destiny. Who am I? What am I doing here? Who are all these others?** Our experiences may have led us to conclude 'I am sick I will never do anything good. Other people are successful'.

The first thing to be decided about your script is whether it is negative or positive. This can be discovered very quickly by listening to what you say. People with positive scripts say things like: 'I made a mistake, but it will not happen again' or 'now I have learned, I will do things differently'. People with negative scripts say for example: 'If only...', 'I can't...', 'Yes but...' The person with the positive script knows what to do, and what action to take if he has a problem The person with the negative script does not know, chooses not to find out or be active around problem solving.

Implications for Change

Teaching script theory is likely to expose the script decisions we have made and therefore offer us relief by enabling us to reconsider the decisions which are controlling our lives. We all, at one time or another, play roles and mark ourselves out in some way. Script theory makes us aware of when we are putting on a performance and this awareness provides the freedom to reject false roles. Play-acting can be given up in favour of authenticity. The range of possible influences contained in **Handout Nine: Considering My Script and Other Questions,** highlight the significance of work on Scripts in discovering why we are who we are!

Summary

Transactional analysis provides a theoretical model of personality, and a therapeutic tool, and therefore can assist in opening the doors for change and new behaviour. However, if any new decisions are to be meaningful they should, according to TA theory, be integrated into all the ego states. Pivotal to TA theory is the belief that early decisions based upon faulty data and illusions about the world can be altered. Transactional Analysis requires that an individual makes a new decision about his world view. **It is the prerogative of the individual to decide the need for these kinds of life changes.**

Moreover, instead of uncovering repressed traumas in the individual's history, TA is aimed at indentifying the illusions governing the individual's present actions. The particular self concept we hold or, in other words, the life position we take. The options that we are able to see, and explore in our life, set the limits to our general 'world view'. Our **life position** sets the plan we will make, and endeavour to fulfil throughout our life.

TA argues that there are four basic life positions. A working knowledge and understanding of TA and life positions will enhance significantly the helper's ability to help.

Life Positions:

Life positions are an essential part of TA theory. **Life positions are based on the conclusions an individual makes about himself and his relation to others.**

☐ **I'm OK – you're OK.** People with this position have a basic realistic acceptance of the importance of other people, including themselves, and they reflect an optimistic and healthy outlook on life. It is the position people need to have in order to achieve their fullest potential. (Many people fail to achieve their potential because of their lack of self-esteem and because of their 'unwillingness' to invest trust in others.)

☐ **I'm OK – you're not OK.** This is the position taken by people who feel victimised or persecuted and consequently they actually victimise and persecute others. People in this position blame others for their misery. They may deny personal difficulties, feel cheated, and react towards the world with anger or frustration. (Some people become so extremely suspicious and cheated by others that they feel justified in robbing, brutalizing, or even killing.)

☐ **I'm not OK – you're OK.** This position is common to people who feel powerless when they compare themselves with others. It is the position which is related to depression, inferiority, inadequacy, guilt, fear, and distrust of others. People in this position are often isolates and, in severe cases, may commit suicide.

☐ **I'm not OK – you're not OK.** This position causes people to feel hopeless and lose interest in living. They may act in a confused way, may be severely depressed, irritated, and behave unpredictably. Neither they, nor anyone else, are worthwhile or valuable. These persons often end up in prisons and mental institutions and they may commit suicide and/or murder to get even or escape from 'life'. (Harris, 1967.)

In summary, **individuals make sense of themselves and the world by developing a subjective map of the objective world,** thus leading them to believe, for example: 'that is what people are like', 'everyone for themselves'. Such views are not just a way of labelling others and events but are a means of 'understanding' and 'predicting' events.

Life positions are established when predictions based on them are validated – 'I failed my exam, now I know I am not OK'.

Discounting and Symbiosis:

Many of the problems people have and much emotional disturbance, including self-concept and life positions, is behaviour learned which results from unresolved symbiotic relationships. **Symbiosis** occurs when two or more individuals behave as though between them they form a whole person.

This relationship is characterised by neither individual utilizing their own ability to feel, think, and behave autonomously. (With reference to TA theory, it would be argued the individual is not using his full complement of ego states.) The psychological mechanism used by people to maintain symbiosis is called 'discounting'. (Schiff, 1975.)

Symbiosis is described as a normal condition in the early stages in the development of the child. It is experienced by both the mother and the child as a merging or sharing of their needs. It is seen as necessary for normal early development and the survival of the child. When symbiosis is impaired in the early months, or prolonged beyond the period of life when the child should be experiencing separation from the mother, emotional disturbance is likely to arise.

Whenever an adult is attempting to establish or maintain a symbiosis beyond the appropriate development stage, he is ignoring or distorting some aspect of the child's internal or external experience. **Discounting preserves the individual's view of the world. There are four levels of discounting, and within these levels a person can discount in three areas, himself, others, and the situation.**

1. **Level One: Discounting the existence of a problem:**

   ☐ **Himself:** "I don't feel angry", said by an angry person
   ☐ **Others:** "He is OK", said by a person watching another being bullied

- **Situation:** "I'm always cared for at home", said by a person who is repeatedly rejected at home

Here we see that the person is reducing the impact of the internal or external stimulus, or message, by selectively denying information or ignoring information directly related to solving the problem. The examples illustrate the thinking pattern involved. Once the person learns more about his patterns of behaving – recognising and acknowledging the discounting of reality – he may begin to correct his thinking and behaviour.

2. Level Two: Discounting the significance of the problem:

- **Himself:** "I'm always angry and it never causes me any problems", said by a person charged with assault
- **Others:** "Being bullied doesn't hurt anymore", said by a person being bullied
- **Situation:** "I don't mind not being wanted", said by a person being rejected

Since the problem is not considered significant, the person places no energy into solving it. This is the use of 'rationalisation' as a defence mechanism invoked as a means of defending a self-concept or life position.

3. Level Three: Discounting the solvability of the person:

- **Himself:** "My father was always angry, I'm just like him, that's the way it is"
- **Others:** "Some people have always been bullied, it cannot be stopped", said by someone watching someone being bullied
- **Situation:** "People like me are always in trouble", said by someone being arrested

There is an awareness of the problem here, but a belief that it cannot be solved.

1. **Level Four: Discounting personal ability to solve the problem:**

☐ **Himself:** "I know people change, but I'll always be angry", said by someone charged with grievous bodily harm

☐ **Others:** "I don't like seeing Bob bully others, but he can't change", said by Bob's friend

☐ **Situation:** "I can't change therefore I will have to face the consequences", said by Bob on his way to prison for the fifth time

From the above it can be seen that the person is involved in getting someone else to solve the problem, while discounting his own ability to problem solve. Discounting maintains the symbiosis as personal responsibility is not being accepted or owned. Discounting is a thinking problem.

In order to establish a symbiotic relationship a person utilizes ways in which he gets other people to think, feel, and solve problems for him. To achieve this he will use passive, non-thinking and non-feeling, behaviours which are seen as resulting from unresolved dependency needs (that is symbiosis), and are the external manifestations of discounting.

Passive Behaviour:

There are four styles of passive behaviour which a person may use to start a symbiotic relationship.

☐ **Doing nothing,** and waiting for someone else to do the thinking, feeling, or doing that a given situation demands. For example, when John observed Robert stealing he sat still and did nothing to intervene or notify others.

☐ **Over-adaptation**, being over-complaint, and viewing others as parent figures who are more important and whose needs and wants are 'my responsibility to figure out and resolve'. For example, John wished for someone to go with him to the shops but would not ask because he assumed that no-one would wish to go with him.

☐ **Agitation,** involves the use of energy in purposeless non-goal-oriented activities. These activities avoid thinking, feeling or problem solving. For example, pacing, hair twisting, finger tapping, talking incessantly, foot tapping and so forth. Mild and even moderate agitation can be alleviated by increasing the person's awareness of it, by identifying the message the agitation is expressing indirectly. For example, 'Just sit still, put your hands upon your knees, no one is going to hurt you'.

☐ **Incapacitation and/or violence,** these behaviours again involve a refusal to think, feel or problem solve and are immediate demands on the environment to take over the responsibility. These behaviours may include becoming sick, aggressive outburst, attacking someone, and so on. All result in the avoidance of autonomy. Passive behaviours indicate discounting in an attempt to establish or maintain a symbiosis.

In helping it is important that the helper knows when and how people establish symbiotic relationships so that the helper does not unwittingly support symbiosis or attempts to establish symbiosis. Confronting the helpee can be as mild as crossing a transaction, refusing to answer a question when the helpee knows the answer, or even giving positive strokes or messages when the helpee is seeking a negative one. Confrontation also includes not responding at all. **The essential quality of a good confrontation is that it thwarts the helpee's attempt to establish a symbiosis and thereby invites the helpee to do something different.**

The helpee will either persist, escalate by discounting more heavily, stop coming to the helping situation and find someone else to be symbiotic with, or accept the invitation to change. The first two possibilities can be confronted still further. Another option may result in the helper establishing a new contract with the helpee with a clause stating: to think about, talk about, and problem solve, the reasons for, and urges associated behind not coming. Or, the helper may need to terminate the arrangements.

If the helper is familiar with TA he would usually confront attempts to establish symbiosis from the same ego state as the one the helpee is using. For example, a person attempting to establish a symbiosis from his Child ego state by inviting the helper into Parent:

Helpee: (from Child ego state) "I just can't face this without you"

Helper: (from Child ego state) "I can't stand it when you act like a baby"

Or, the helper could report from his Adult ego state on how his Child ego state is feeling, "I hear you. I think you want something from me. It is true?"

However, if the person is attempting to establish symbiosis from Parent ego state the helper could respond as follows:

Helpee: (from Parent ego state) "You should take more care of me and give me more attention"

Helper: (from his Parent ego state) "I experience that you are 'acting' silly; tell me how you feel"

For assessing the level and frequency of symbiosis and passive behaviours the following check list offers a guide:

☐ **Symbiosis:** does the person use all his ego states to solve problems? Which ego state does he use? Which ego states are not used?

☐ **Passive Behaviours:** is the person actively seeking a solution to his problems? Does he agitate instead of thinking, instead of feeling? Does he incapacitate himself in any way, headaches, illness, etc? Is he violent to self or others? Is he pleasing himself or others?

There are two further processes which people use in order to avoid resolving problems or behaving autonomously. They are: 'redefining transactions' and 'grandiosity'.

79

Redefining Transactions occurs whenever someone discounts some aspect of communication, and shifts the issues in order to maintain an established view.

Helper: "What time does your bus leave?"

Helpee: "Can you come with me?"

Here the shift is from the request for information to, You. Redefining disallows the question or stimulus be altering its meaning.

Helper: "Do you understand the point I am making?"

Helpee: "Do you mind if I close the window?"

Here the shift is away from responding to the question, with the helpee asking a completely unrelated question. Redefining is an attempt to control, and also to avoid dealing with issues.

Grandiosity involves an exaggeration (maximization or minimalization) of some aspect of self, others, or the situation. Grandiosity compensates for the individual's perception of themselves as inadequate. (Schiff, 1975.) Examples of grandiose words and expressions will be:

'...fantastic, always, never, can't help it, can't stand it and superlatives like best, worst, least ...' and so on.

The thinking underlying grandiosity affects a shift of responsibility to others and/or the situation.

Helper: "Peter, would you be good enough to make a cup of tea?"

Helpee: "I can't stand making tea"

Grandiose words need to be confronted and a meaningful definition sought so that a complete understanding from the helper's point of view is achieved, in other words, encouraging the helpee to make statements that are concrete.

Helper: "What feelings do you have?"

Helpee: "I always feel helpless"

Here the helper will need to explore what is meant by 'always' and what is meant by 'helpless'. He could ask for an explanation of what 'always' means in terms of a time measure or ask 'when do you feel competent?' The helper may choose to ask 'why are you allowing yourself to feel scared (or angry, or sad)?'

Discounting, passive behaviours, redefining, and grandiosity are mechanisms used, often outside of awareness of their consequences, so as to maintain a life position and avoid goal directed or problem-solving behaviour.

Frequently, problems and the source of conflict, is in the lack of a clear perception of alternatives on the part of the helpee. The anxiety that problems cause is clearly unpleasant and often results in ill-defined feelings of apprehension occurring in situations in which the helpee feels threatened. All work in helping must be based upon the intrinsic worth and value of the helpee. This means the helper does not consider the helpee to be inadequate, defective, or incapable of change, no matter what the 'diagnosis'. On the other hand, this does not mean that the helper and the helpee just smile benignly at whatever the helpee does or says. The helper maintains a positive view of the helpee even though the helper may feel and verbalise concern about the helpee's behaviour. Remember, 'what we once decided to do can be re-decided'. **When the helper confronts behaviour he assumes the responsibility to communicate information in such a way that he does not imply to the helpee that he is somehow 'bad'.**

CHAPTER FIVE

Am I Going Mad?

So far we have endeavoured to consider material which will assist us in understanding our own psychology and the psychology of others. We are beginning to see how difficult it is to understand why another person behaves in a particular way and also, sometimes, how difficult it is to understand why we ourselves feel and behave the way we do! Acquiring insight and awareness into what might be considered the 'normal range' of behaviour is difficult enough and we can see it requires our full attention, thought and energy.

Behaviour beyond the 'normal range' is far more perplexing to comprehend. Much helping or counselling is relatively routine and deals with the range of problems most of us encounter, albeit at different degrees of intensity, throughout our lives. 'I have lost any sense of direction in my life, especially now the children have grown up' is something many of us will experience. However, horrifying incidents of unusual behaviour, for example, extreme acts of violence, or child murder, find us saying things like, 'he's a mental case'.

The helper has responsibility to acquaint himself with the symptoms of abnormal behaviour so that he is better placed to recognise its existence, seek guidance, or support, or refer to a more experienced clinician. The complexity of the management and treatment of abnormal behaviour requires the concerted effort of all. The skilled and aware helper will recognise symptoms or problems which are beyond his capabilities, and it is not his role to engage in the desperate struggle to keep people from going insane.

We have considered some of the factors that promote self-growth and self-actualization and, therefore, by implication understand more clearly forces that impede growth. However, much less is known about how behaviour becomes so distorted and distant from what most of us would understand as normal, and how such distortion might be prevented, or treated, in order to halt acceleration.

The ability of most helpers to judge the severity of the various symptoms found in abnormal behaviour will, it is suggested, be limited. For a helper to say someone is 'mental' is no more or less useful, than to say someone is 'physical'. Labelling is extremely dangerous and it can be of no surprise that the person labelled as 'inadequate' often becomes inadequate. It is equally extremely dangerous to use in helping inaccurate and poorly understood terms and phrases. The helper must be extremely disciplined in the language he uses and the messages he transmits.

The helper's role in respect to the overall well-being of the helpee is crucial for he is responsible for the emotional tone, sensitivity, and integrity of the helping environment, that is, if the helpee is not to be cheated!

Sometimes, when people are facing specific traumas or are in difficulty with themselves, their lives, relationships, or other issues which have led them to seek help, they will often speak of a fear of losing control, becoming out of control, or their mind becoming deranged. 'Am I going mad?', 'Will I end up in a psychiatric hospital?' are the questions often asked. Thankfully, it is usually possible to reassure most people. The idea of the mind, however, is a nebulous one. It is part religious and part philosophical.

When we speak of diseases of the mind we are speaking more realistically of diseases which create a disturbance in the brain or central nervous system and the way in which these systems function. The mind, as distinct from the purely religious concept of the soul, refers to the manifestation or function of the brain – it is the way the brain works at a conscious and subconscious level. **The mind embraces the total personality** – the character, intellect, and emotion, the thinking, and behaviour of an individual. Yet the mind functions through chemicals and electrical impulses. Few would now argue about the interrelationship between the body and the mind and that neither operates in isolation from the other or in isolation from wider environmental, sociological, biological, or psychological influences. Although the causation of abnormal behaviour remains the subject of scientific study certain conditions have been classified.

Although there are numerous books on the subject of abnormal behaviour and dictionaries explaining particular terms, a short definition is provided here for those terms which are used, usually inappropriately, in our everyday language particularly when we are making allusions to, or descriptions of, certain behaviours.

One of the main subdivisions within the arena of mental health is that of psychosis and neurosis.

☐   psychosis refers to a severe form of mental illness in which insight is lost. That is, the individual ceases to be aware of the disturbance in their thinking or emotion - which is clearly apparent to an outside observer – and they interpret their thinking, emotion, attitude, and behaviour as being an appropriate response to their environment. Thus, patients with a psychotic depression do come to believe 'that the sins of the world are really upon them'. Schizophrenia is an example of a psychotic illness

☐   neurosis is a condition in which insight is retained and this is true even in the severest forms of such conditions. Anxiety states, obsessional states, and phobias would be examples of neuroses

Other terms frequently used:

☐   delusion is a false belief that is held with conviction and contrary to the individual's upbringing and cultural background and not amenable to reasoned argument. For example, lightening being a demonstration that the Gods are unhappy

☐   hallucination is a false perception in the absence of external stimulus. Thus the individual who hears a voice, which no one else can hear, seemingly coming from inside his head, or from somewhere outside and nearby, is said to be hallucinating. Such perceptions arise within the individual's central nervous system but they are perceived by the person

84

not as his own thoughts or memories but are in some way coming from outside. Hallucinations may affect sight, smell, taste, or touch

☐ illusion in contrast, is a mistake or misinterpreted perception. Here an individual perceives something through one of his senses but makes an error or perception in interpreting this data. For example, he is convinced that the shadow in the bushes was man lurking in the bushes

☐ paranoia refers to abnormal suspiciousness. For example, 'I know (and said with real conviction) everyone is after me'

The above conditions require most careful diagnosis and the damage that such inappropriate diagnosis can do is sobering to contemplate!

It has been acknowledged that the functions of the body and mind are inextricably linked. Often helpees will describe physical conditions or illnesses and although not necessarily the province of the helper, an awareness of psychosomatic disorders can only be helpful.

Psychosomatic Disorders:

Psychosomatic disorders are attributed in part to the external state of the individual. The most obvious difference between them is the part of the body affected. The reason why one particular organ or part of the body suffers is unknown and continues to be an area of study. As psychosomatic disorders are real diseases involving damage to the body and the fact that they are caused by emotional factors does not make the affliction imaginary. People can just as readily die from psychosomatic disorders (asthma/ulcers) as from infection or physical injury. Parts of the body affected include:

☐ the skin: for example, inflammation, itching, dryness, eczema

☐ respiration: for example, asthma, hay-fever, sighing, hiccoughs, breathing very rapidly

- cardio-vascular system: for example, heart racing, high blood pressure, blushing

- gastro-intestinal system: for example, ulcers, acidity, heartburn, constipation

- genital urinary system: for example, disturbances in menstruation and urination, urinary frequency, impotence.

- muscular skeletal system: for example, backache, cramps, tension headaches

In addition to the above, many other diseases are viewed as being partially caused by emotional or psychological factors, for example, multiple sclerosis, pneumonia, cancer, and the common cold. In short, the emotional state of the individual is recognised as playing a critical role in illness. Put at its most simple – 'I feel happy, I am well,' 'I feel unhappy, I am sick'.

In summary, all functioning and all diseases are both mental and physical as both elements are going on continuously and strongly suggests we are looking at a monistic system rather that a dualistic one. It is for the biologically and psychologically orientated theorists to explain why only some people develop given symptoms and what determines the particular symptom or disorder?

It is important to remind ourselves that a **healthy body and mind** cannot function on junk food. Hence **good nutrition** is essential if good mental and physical health is to be achieved and then maintained. Good health cannot be taken for granted and we have to take personal responsibility for it. Our diet and health care routines are key aspects of our self-image, life position, and script. Dietary change may be a primary issue in the change process. **(See: We are also what we eat)**

Suicide:

One thing that is guaranteed to shock most of us is to hear that someone close to us has committed suicide. It is not unusual for certain helpees to say 'I feel like killing myself'. The helper, as emphasised earlier in the book, is not responsible for the helpee's behaviour – remember we each **own our own behaviour**. The earlier discussion on the discounting and symbiosis provides a useful framework for the helper in addressing this issue. It is worth being aware of at least some of the facts. Two types of suicidal acts may be distinguished:

- a serious intent to produce death where careful plans are made and in such cases attempts to commit suicide are often successful

- suicidal gestures (known as parasuicide) involving for example, overdoses or self mutilation, occur but do not usually produce death. This is not to assume there is a clear dividing line between the serious intent and the accident. Parasuicide is more than ten times as common as the first and successful suicide is more common in men than in women. This is in contrast to parasuicide which is commoner in women

The range of facts known about self-intentioned death assists us in appreciating how complex this issue is:

- the commonest method of self-intentioned death is self-poisoning – the overdose

- three times as many men kill themselves as women

- three times as many women as men attempt to kill themselves but do not die

- suicide is found in both the old and the young – even below ten years of age

- suicide is found almost equally at all social and economic levels, and

- no other form of death leaves friends and relatives with such long-lasting feelings of distress and general disturbance

A range of theories exist about suicide, for example, aggression turned inwards, retaliation by inducing guilt in others, efforts to make amends for perceived past wrongs, efforts to rid oneself of unacceptable feelings or escape from stress, and the desire to rejoin a dead loved one.

Our current understanding of these theories or explanations remains questionable but it is possible to comment on a number of prevalent **misconceptions and myths about suicide**:

- 'People who discuss suicide will not commit suicide' – the fact is that up to three-quarters of those who take their lives have communicated the intent beforehand

- 'People commit suicide without warning' – the falseness of this belief is indicated in the preceding statement. There seem to be many warnings such as person saying 'the world would be better off without me', etc.

- 'It is only people of a certain class that commit suicide' – suicide is neither a blight of the poor or a curse on the rich. People of all classes commit suicide

- 'It is easy to establish the motives for suicide' – the truth is there is only the poorest understanding of why people commit suicide and why individuals differ in the reactions to seemingly similar sets of social conditions

- 'Most of the people that commit suicide are depressed' – this myth does not account for the tragic fact that signs of the impending suicide are overlooked in people who are not depressed people, who do at some time think of or attempt suicide

- 'People who commit suicide must be insane' – although many suicidal persons may be unhappy, most do appear to be completely rational and in touch with reality

- 'The tendency to commit suicide is inherited' – there is no evidence to support this

- 'Suicide in some people is caused by the weather or the moon' – there is no evidence to support such belief

- 'People who commit suicide clearly want to die' – most people who commit suicide appear to be ambivalent about their own deaths

With reference to the material of this chapter and the old adage 'there is only one thing guaranteed in life and that's death' the effective helper needs to have worked out for himself, and understand for himself, how the reality of death affects him so that he is more able to deal with bereavement issues and fear of death in others.

Thou Shall Surely Die:

Many of the people seeking help, and in particular those who may be unwell, or where there is serious illness in the family, will be thinking of, or worrying about, dying. Despite the statement 'thou shall surely die' many people live their lives as if they believe themselves to be immortal! It seems that at least one of the paradoxes for mankind is that he knows he is unique in nature (with consciousness and imagination) yet he is also food for the worms.

We know that even during the most pleasant days, the fate of death is ever present. Man submits himself to a 'social reality' and plays it safe in the world. He is practised at self-deceit for although he knows he is not immortal few understand for themselves, or prepare for that ultimate reality.

One of the Sigmund Freud's major discoveries was that psychological illness is the fear of knowledge of oneself, of one's emotions, impulses, memories, and potentialities, of one's destiny.

Many of us in fact live, as the Danish philosopher Soren Kierkegaard put it, 'by tranquillising themselves with the trivial'. The reality of death can be lied about by tricks of deception and repression, but the anxiety produced cannot be lied about. By facing up to the anxiety, the lie is destroyed.

Clearly some students of helping, helpers and helpees, will hold personally satisfying religious or philosophical beliefs. It is only when we begin to consider our beliefs, feelings, and their relationship, to not only our own death but our life, will we decide for ourselves our own position on such ultimate questions.

It is unacceptable for a helper to say, 'I don't wish to speak about death' and it is equally unacceptable for a helper to impose his beliefs on the helpee.

Advice giving, for example, 'If I were you I wouldn't worry about what you are worrying about' or 'The answer to your problem is my belief system' is the worst possible form of helping as it totally negates the helpee's own capacity to think, behave, and resolve to his own satisfaction, such issues. This is not to say that discussion on the subject should be avoided, on the contrary, it is as valid as any other subject in helping, but must be approached from the principles which inform good practice, and in particular, **enabling the helpee to find his own helper within himself.**

The helper acts as a sounding board and sometimes as a 'vessel' for the helpee's feelings. The feelings of others, like fear of death, can arouse fear of death in us. Two factors determine how effective a helper will be as a 'vessel or container' for the helpee's feelings:

☐ his own strength in terms of his own self-awareness and knowledge of the source and meaning of his own feelings, and

☐ the pressure of the 'contents' of the feelings, be they the ones expressed by the helpee, or the ones held by the helper

Again, it cannot be over-emphasised, that is, the requirement of the helper to be involved in his own development and self-understanding. People who are genuinely able to work their way through their own painful feelings to a 'peace of mind' can be thought to be strong enough 'containers' to hold potentially overwhelming feelings from others, and help others in making such feelings safe. It is interesting to note, that when we hold

90

powerful or distressing feelings inside, we often **feel as if we are disintegrating or breaking-up!**

Therefore, our own personal work, and work with prospective helpers, cannot avoid the ultimate questions, as they will arise in helping others. These can be approached in a structured way and the following questions may offer direction.

- What is the greatest fear now?

- Do you face the future with hope or fear?

- What does your treasure consist of?

- Do you anticipate death as a release or as a next step or...?

- Are you willing to imagine your own death and write a brief and objective obituary of yourself?

It has been argued that we live, consciously or unconsciously with a death wish, and, alternatively, it has been claimed that the main problem facing human beings is a fear of embracing the overwhelming wonder of life... each position, of course, is dependent upon a given view of the world, a given self-concept! The aim of exploring questions, like those above, is to establish with greater clarity what our views and the views of clients may be.

When confronted with the unknown, most people are likely to be anxious, or even fearful. This is common and applies to many situations, including approaching death. Fear of death itself is perhaps less common than expected (although younger people are likely to think they were cheated if death comes early). Older people can be remarkably phlegmatic about death – 'I am 85 years old, I've had a good life and am now ready to go'. As already stated, the helper needs to have established his own position on the question of death. Is it total extinction? Is there something beyond death that gives it meaning? These are timeless questions which have been discussed at various intellectual levels down the ages. The religious perspective cannot be denied and I suggest it is also worth considering further some of the psychological perceptions on this subject.

Vicktor Frankel (1959) was an existential psychotherapist. He formulated his theories in a Nazi concentration camp where, as a fellow victim, he saw thousands die. His basic tenet is that people can endure the most appalling difficulties and hardships provided they can find meaning in the situation. He was fond of quoting Friedrich Nietzsche: 'He who has a why to live can endure almost any how'. According to Frankel, the primary motivating force in man is the search for meaning. He called it 'the will to meaning' in contrast to the 'will to pleasure', on which Freudian psychoanalysis is based, or the 'will to power' stressed the psychologist, Alfred Adler. Despite the importance Frankel gives to meaning, he makes no generalisation about life or death. For him the significance of life or death differs from person to person and from day to day.

What matters is not the general but the specific meaning, at any given moment, for any one person, and the level of pressure or responsibility with which any given challenge makes, as accepted or rejected by that person, at that given moment.

Carl Jung (1986) advocated a positive attitude to death. He finds it in accord with the collective psyche of humanity to regard death as the fulfilment of life's meaning, and its goal, in its truest sense. He considers those who see death as a meaningless cessation to life, to have isolated them psychologically, and therefore they stand opposed to their own basic human nature. Jung considers the psyche begins its preparation for death in middle life, and that dying has its onset before death. He expresses astonishment at how little concern the psyche makes of death as an event, but he believed the unconscious 'is really interested in how one dies', that is whether the attitude of the conscious mind is adjusted to dying or not. In this he seems to be in agreement with Frankel.

Bereavement:

Whatever views the helper holds he will know that the majority of people die in hospital but most of the grieving will take place at home. The time of bereavement is a crisis in the person's life but it can be a time of personal growth as a new but different life is found.

The helper must be aware of his own emotional responses when dealing with dying and death and use his skills, communication and understanding, to provide the highest possible level of support. He will make time to:

☐ listen and be sensitive to the patient's feelings and inner needs

☐ facilitate discussion of anxieties, fears and suspicions regarding possible guilt and irrational fears

☐ be as optimistic as the situation permits to avoid any sense of hopelessness, and

☐ explain and offer support in the process of bereavement and grieving

Grieving is a natural process through which many people progress using their own resources, and usually with the help and support of family and friends. During the state of numbness and disbelief, which may happen immediately after the death and last for several hours or days, it may be necessary to prompt the bereaved relative to talk about their loved one in order to start the process of grieving. Often, the newly bereaved person feels the urge to cry out, to search and try and find the person who has died. There may be anger and irritability with the helper. Intense feelings of guilt may arise – 'could have done more for him'. A period of apathy and depression may follow.

The most useful thing the helper can do is sit and listen. There is usually an outpouring of emotions and feelings.

Bereaved people may need to be reassured that they are not going 'mad', and what they are experiencing is normal, even though it is very painful. Hasty decisions can be made during bereavement, for example, moving house. This can be disastrous and serve only to prolong the grieving process. The bereaved person should be invited to reconsider major decisions and wait until their lives become more settled. Clearly, absence of grief – in situations when it would normally be expected – should be taken as a sign that all is not going as it should. In such a situation the helper will invite the bereaved person to consider more fully his feelings and if necessary refer to a more skilled clinician.

Normal bereavement involves a sense of numbness which can last for a few days. At this time shock and disbelief act as a defence as the bereaved person tries to deal with the reality of the death. There may be episodes of severe distress and at other times little sign of outward emotion. However, as the reality of the loss begins to be absorbed, the grief becomes more prominent. As the feelings of numbness fade, the pain of grieving increases, there may be a need to search for the dead person and this searching, accompanied by crying, is seen as pining and preoccupation with thoughts of the dead person. However, as the searching continues without result, feelings of helplessness and anxiety may increase. Anger is often expressed at the dead person or at the helper. Anger may also be shown towards 'God' and the bereaved often go over and over the events surrounding the death trying to make sense of what happened.

Guilt may be felt, especially if there has been disharmony before the death, for example, the wife whose husband left home to go to work following a row and suddenly dies. Moreover, if it has been an ambivalent relationship, guilt may then be pronounced. Many unresolved conflicts may exist, even an unexpressed death wish which has now come to fruition. As grief deepens, anxiety increases and associated physical sensations like tightness in the chest and breathlessness may follow. Agitation and restlessness are common in an aim to reduce and cope with the feelings of grief and many varying stimuli act as triggers for grief, such as hearing a favourite tune or meeting with a sympathetic friend.

With time there is a gradual lessening of the feelings of acute grief although feelings of despair and depression may follow. The bereaved may become socially isolated as they become disinterested in everything around them. This may continue for many months until there is a gradual acceptance of the loss, and the acceptance of new roles. A new identity is developed as roles which were once those of the dead person are taken on and self-esteem is strengthened.

These stages are not clear cut and there is no straightforward progression from one to another. Pangs of grief may be felt many months or years after the death – perhaps as a memory is stimulated. However, with time most bereaved people are able to 'live again', although altered by the experience of loss.

It is clear that the role for the helper, and his skills, can make a significant contribution through the process of bereavement, grief, and the 'recovery' which follows.

True Insight:

Our life is a challenge to growth. We have talked about 'wholeness' in terms of an increased awareness which harmonizes our thoughts, feelings, behaviour, and we have acknowledged that is by improving our understanding of these functions of our personality, that true personal insight and growth becomes possible. Not only does this imply growth in terms of how we relate to ourselves and our world, it further implies that there is a state of 'Enlightenment' that this is attainable by all, and that there is a method or processes available for the attainment of Enlightenment... the peak of self-actualization.

- enlightenment – is beyond the 'ego mind', which is influenced by desire, is separate from the outer world, which creates a 'dualistic' view of life – 'I and others' – which is the cause of discord and suffering and is therefore contrary to the harmonious way of nature and is fundamentally illusion. 'I' is an idea formed in our mind and is not the truth of our reality. Enlightenment is attained by recovering the 'pure' truth of our reality. The essence of enlightenment arises from knowing the true nature of all things. By removing from the mind feelings of unhappiness and happiness – the source of our suffering – the mind is left peaceful and is able to perceive things as they really are, that is, a pure life force in everything and always present. The mind of 'ignorance' sees things as dualistic, is based upon reasoning, and therefore contains illusion. The 'ignorant' mind sees, for example, a tree which in fact is the idea of a tree and is not a tree itself. The tree, or the field, or the gate, are ideas and not pure reality.

☐   pure reality is contained in all things and it is this that the Enlightenment mind can see. At the point of Enlightenment there is no tree, no field, and no gate, just pure reality or empty mind. The enlightened mind is of course able to perceive pure reality contained within the tree and the whole universe. The insight which Enlightenment offers is not to create a system of beliefs but rather to show how to see clearly into the nature of the mind and the nature of all things. Such insight and the Enlightenment which follows gives rise to a sense of deep calm which is beyond superficial knowledge, showing that everything is related in a pure 'Oneness'.

Enlightenment can be obtained by each of us – throughout history the existence of this state of Enlightenment has been confirmed, most notably by the Buddha. Enlightenment is therefore available to all who are participating fully in their own growth and ultimately progress beyond the notion of 'self' with the realisation that there is no permanent self. Therefore, Enlightenment is attainable for all involving a level of insight which will allow even unpleasant experiences to be insightful.

By looking clearly at our attitudes, intentions, and desires, we can investigate the relationship between each and the unpleasant experiences and dissatisfaction which often result. By increasing our insight we become clearer about the ideas and thoughts which come and go through the mind, see thoughts and ideas for what they really are, and begin to leave the mind clear and refreshed.

Such is the ongoing path of insight. To be able to go to a still centre of awareness in the mind, bring awareness into our life, and thereby live peacefully with the variety of feelings that arise in our consciousness is indeed a worthwhile journey.

One process or method for attaining Enlightenment is meditation. Meditation is not a goal in itself but a proven method which allows us to attain a silence of our mind, and thus enter a pure state of consciousness or Enlightenment.

You need to find a time and place which affords you calm and freedom from disturbance and the ideal posture is sitting in an upright position with your back straight. Be mindful of your posture and check to see if your body is holding any tension and quietly allow the muscles to relax. You can sit on the floor with your legs crossed with a small cushion at the back of the buttocks to support the angle of your hips, or you may choose to sit in an upright chair. Allow the chin to tilt slightly forwards to ensure that the spine is straight and place your hands on your lap, palms upward, one gently resting on the other with the thumb tips touching. Gather your attention, be aware of your body, relax any tensions – particularly in the face and neck – and allow your eyelids to close. Meditation is effortless.

You sit in stillness and allow your mind to become aware of the inhalation and exhalation of the breath. The mind will wander but just quietly bring your attention back to your breath. You will be aware of your breath filling your chest and the abdomen. You will notice the workings of the mind as thoughts come and go. Just simply and effortlessly bring attention back to the breath.

The entire process can be summarised as follows:

☐ gathering your attention by focusing on your posture

☐ noticing and focusing upon your breath

☐ noticing that the mind has wandered, and

☐ re-establishing your attention on the breath

There are other forms of meditation available and these will range from walking meditation to the use of a mantra (a word or sound repeated out loud or within the mind), but it must be emphasised that whatever method of meditation you choose, meditation is a method for achieving that goal of Enlightenment, and Enlightenment can only be achieved by 'letting go' within meditation and therefore, paradoxically seeking no goal. With meditation our insight deepens and we can begin to see more clearly the results of our thoughts, feelings, and behaviours. With increased insight greater sensitivity follows and we are able to observe the distress we cause ourselves and others, and this will often inspire us to wish to live more wisely. Meditation, when combined with a commitment to personal responsibility, will encourage us to care for ourselves and others in a more meaningful way.

There is nothing mysterious about gaining the insight that leads to Enlightenment. In the words of the Buddha, the way is simple – 'do good, refrain from doing evil, and purify the mind'!

Beside what you think, feel and do, you are also what you eat.

We Are Also What We Eat:

As we each become more self aware and are therefore developing our 'whole person' it usually follows that we consider or reconsider what we actually eat. Once we acknowledge the inter-relationship between what we eat, the biochemical balance of our body, our health, and also our attitudes, values, and behaviour – which are in part linked to our diet – we begin to realise more fully we are also what we eat!

Diet then, is a most valid issue for the helper to explore the helpee.

Initially, in most cases, diet will be a 'lower' order of priority to that of more 'major' presenting problems. However, what is true is that to ensure a clear mind and healthy body a balanced diet is critical. Moreover, a change of diet often precedes a change of lifestyle, a change of lifestyle implies the giving up of old behaviours and habits, and is therefore part of becoming.

In this context, such becoming is likely to involve the individual in developing a more holistic lifestyle. He will become more aware of environmental issues such as pollution; Green issues such as the protection of the forests; as well as the implications of how food is produced, particularly in terms of ecology. For example:

- it takes three pounds of grain to produce one pound of poultry, or, ten pounds of grain to produce one pound of beef

- In oriental countries 90% of cereal crop is consumed directly as food. In Britain and Western Europe only 30% and in North America only 14% is consumed directly

- on average, an acre of land used for grain production gives five times as much protein as an acre used for producing meat, and

- an acre of beans or lentils give ten times as much protein as meat, and an acre of vegetables 15 times as much protein

When dealing with diet the helper is dealing with the whole person not just an enquiry into what the helpee eats. A diet history will reveal an enormous amount about the psychology of the helpee. Diet is therefore an important diagnostic tool, for example:

The excessive consumption of fruit may produce someone who is flighty and inconsistent; he will be calmed down by eating brown rice and boiled vegetables. Eating excess quantities of red meat creates aggression and bad temper. Vegetarians are usually more placid and peaceful.

A healthy diet is a balanced diet. A balance of cooked and raw foods, with an ideal intake of vitamins, proteins, carbohydrates, water and fats, plus, sufficient intake of fibre to ensure good bowel function. Keep the intake of salt and sugar (along with artificial additives of all descriptions) at an absolute minimum. (Knight, 2010)

The importance of diet with regard to helping is that it links into the helping process in a number of ways.

Diet links to:

☐   attitudes and values – 'I will stop eating meat as meat production in uneconomic and also environmentally disastrous in terms of producing protein'. (It has been argued, that the fear and anger an animal experiences in the slaughterhouse stays within the animal's body and that fear and anger is later consumed and absorbed by us, and results in aggressive behaviour)

☐   responsibility for self-care – 'I will be more mindful of what I eat as I realise my behaviour can be affected by my diet and, I realise my health is also affected by my diet.

☐   self-concept – 'Changing, giving up old behaviours, also includes considering diet and I am now beginning to perceive myself as part of a complex ecological system'

Clearly, discussion around diet focuses on the body and acts as a balance between what might be considered the more psychologically based exploration of feelings, thoughts, and behaviours. Moreover, outcomes which follow dietary considerations allow the opportunity for the helpee to take, if he chooses, immediate responsibility for self-care – selecting and administering his own 'prescription' in terms of the food he chooses to eat.

CHAPTER SIX

Discovering Others

The success of the helping relationship depends on the performance of the helper – how well he uses his intuitions, his training, and how well he is able to relate to the helpee. Helpers are in a difficult position in that they aim to encourage helpees of widely different abilities, insights, and motivation to perform to the best of their ability. Clearly, helpers familiar with principles of motivation, of individual difference, and their implications for the achieving change, the helper may also need to be ingenious in vitalising some helpees in terms of confidence and security. Helper competence is fundamental to any consideration of effectiveness in fulfilling the helping task and in doing so will take the helper will responsibility for:

☐ observing the code of ethics

☐ informing the helpee of methods and principles to be used, as well as the duration of sessions and fees (if any)

☐ exploring with the helpee their own expectations of what is involved

☐ confirming with the helpee whether or not they are currently involved in other helping relationships and, if yes and if appropriate, will gain the helpee's permission before conferring with said other professionals

☐ taking account of their own competence, and making alternative referrals when necessary

☐ terminating helping when the helpee has received the help sought, or when it is apparent that help is no longer helping

☐ increasing their own professional development, and also monitoring the limits of their competence

- being actively involved in developing their sense of 'wholeness'

- approaching helping from a position of humility with the understanding that each of us has need – the person being helped and the person helping, and

- recognising that the helpee also has strengths and being aware of this fact

The philosophy informing the helping process discussed in this book is based upon the seminal work of Jacki Lee Schiff at the Cathexis Institute (USA) and the early beginnings and development of that philosophy is described in the 'Cathexis Reader', (1975).

The philosophy takes account of the fact that thinking, feeling, and behaviour problems are usually learned, and do not just happen genetically, or, as a disease process like infection.

The Philosophy Informing Helping:

- the belief that people who have psychological or personal problems are capable of participating in their own change programme

- on some level, people know what they need to do in order to resolve personal difficulties or conflicts

- that all transactions between the helper and the helpee are a part of the helping process

- that inappropriate behaviour is confronted within the 'here and now', and

- that confrontation is equal to caring and being passive is equal to not caring

Problem Solving:

The majority of people seeking, advice, and guidance, are not ill but are in fact, in the main, individuals requiring support in the process of growing, coping, and living.

Change is often conceived of pain and turmoil and arises from present behaviours no longer satisfying. We know that some people prefer their 'misery' to the insecurity which is associated with change. Nevertheless, despair and misery provide the opportunity for personal growth. Growth is unending and inevitable, beginning again and again. Personal development invariably involves pain and difficulty.

The development of our personality is the most personally demanding aspect of our lives. The removal of barriers, delusions, and psychological games are factors fundamental to the growth process. The aim of the helper is therefore to create the situation where the helpee no longer requires him. This will be achieved by affording people the opportunity to discuss freely their life and experience in order to enable that to reclaim their life in a more satisfying and rewarding way. This will, in part, be achieved by the helper developing a climate in which people feel relaxed, are able to be direct and open, and therefore prepared to take a risk in terms of meaningful self disclosure.

Therefore, the one element that is central to the helping relationship is the notion of 'saying things which are normally left unsaid'.

The Aim of Helping:

- to help people solve their immediate problem

- to assist people in developing their own ability to cope with future problems, and

- to help develop new and better ways doing both these things

Specific issues within the helping relationship will invariably contain emotional discomfort and sometimes trauma, but it must be remembered it is often the presence of 'pain' that has initiated the search for help.

Moreover, it must also be remembered that the helper's role is situationally defined and is therefore interchangeable. In other words, **for anyone to look at any other individual and conclude that they are without any personal difficulty indicates one thing only, the other individual is being looked at from the outside.** To look inward would show that their life is similar to ours and that all of us experience a mixture of joy, doubt, conflict, uncertainty, disappointment, sadness, and so on. Sheldon Kopp (1986) captures this reality as follows:

"When a psychotherapy patient does do the work and faces up to some of what he must endure, he is often rewarded by the sense of increased freedom and joy. However, as he comes to realise that there will be no light without some darkness, no rest without toil, he may baulk disappointedly to find troubles never end. New solutions lead to new problems. New freedom leads to new responsibilities".

Self-growth, therefore, will not provide perfection but rather allow us to accept out imperfection more easily by involving greater emphasis on flexibility in our approach to life, and upon gaining greater insight.

Problem solving then is an aspect of learning similar in nature to other forms of learning. The difference basically is one of degree and emphasis rather than of kind. In addition to the resolution of a particular presenting problem, secondary benefits are possible for the helpee:

☐ developing for himself the capacity to identify and initiate his own problem-solving methods

☐ developing his problem solving options is testable ways

☐ experiencing and learning how to discuss problem issues with others

☐ using experience gained through the helping relationship in order to enable him to become a more effective helper for himself

Primary determinants or measures of whether or not an individual is growing towards adequacy and fulfilment is the way in which he responds to experiences and new opportunities.

Of interest in this connection is the **concept of willpower.** Willpower is often used to explain behaviour and in particular in relation to problem solving and growth.

The person who gives up, for example, excessive drinking is said to exercise willpower. The person who fails is said to be lacking in willpower. To attribute differences in willpower is meaningless and fails to acknowledge the factors that promote behaviour.

All behaviour is governed according to a pre-potency of motives and values. Different people have different dominant values and, therefore, different goals, which they strive to obtain with equal compulsion, be they in the area of behaviour, moral conduct, or self-respect.

It is, of course, possible to change dominant values to the point of avoiding or altering previous behaviours but this is no increasing willpower, it is simply substituting new values of a 'higher' level of personal (or social) acceptability.

The excessive drinker, the teacher, the helper, the thief, the Chief Constable, all have essentially the same needs, and each is striving to maintain his world view or self-image intact. They display different behaviours because they have different dominant values. In other words we perceive, interpret, accept, or reject whatever we meet in the light of our own self-system or values – not willpower!

In the quest for growth and the resolution of problems, three questions require to be answered 'Yes' for any action in this area to have any chance of success:

☐ Do you believe the resolution of this problem/s will help you to live and grow more effectively?

☐ Knowing that the resolution of the problem/s will require you facing aspects of yourself and possibly 'buried' issues, are you prepared to proceed?

☐ Are you willing to spend time starting to work on this problem/s?

The Problem-Solving Process:

A useful and proven guide in the process of problem solving is the use of a problem-solving model. The model presented in the following assumes that it is necessary to start with a thorough analysis of the problem.

Problem solving cannot take place without a problem! John Dewey (1930) defines a problem as a 'felt need', which therefore implies that what constitutes a problem for one person may not be a problem for another. Therefore, problem-solving behaviour is initiated not by the existence of a problem in an objective sense, but rather by recognising a particular issue as a problem situation by the given individual.

The problem-solving model is presented as a series of unfolding stage (Knight 1984). The **four stages proposed embrace the core elements** of the majority of existing problem solving models. (Other writers suggest additional steps to the four steps presented here, for example Egan, 1975; Hogwood and Gunn, 1982).

The four stages are as follows:

☐ Problem Diagnosis

☐ Solution Generation

☐ Implementation of Solution

☐ Review

There will be a recurring process going on.

It needs to be borne in mind that a critical fault in all forms of problem solving is that individuals are prone to jump towards a remedy before the particular problem has been sufficiently explored or understood. A meaningful solution would depend upon a through diagnosis of the problem.

The use of a model suggests the process is more or less self-contained and comprises a neat cycle of initial and culminating events. In practice, of course, the process operates within an often bewildering mesh of thoughts, feelings, and behaviours.

The model, when used effectively, acts as an aid to thinking by providing a logical stage by stage approach. Movement, back and forth, means the opportunity for feedback will be possible at each point in the process. The helper therefore uses the model as a logical framework in order to enable him as helper to:

'....relate and respond to the helpee so that the helpee is assisted in exploring his thoughts, feelings, and behaviour so he may cope more effectively with his life by making new and appropriate decisions in accordance with improved self understanding....'

Having a problem implies having at least some information on the subject otherwise the 'problem' would be outside of the helpee's awareness. Nevertheless, the helping process aims to supplement the helpee's knowledge of the problem by further clarification of the problem area. The investigation of the problem will include attempts to break down the problem into more manageable parts.

A simple and proven technique for accomplishing this is the following:

☐ What is the problem?

☐ When does it occur?

☐ Who does it affect?

☐　　Where does it happen?

☐　　Why does it happen?

☐　　How are you (and others) responding, and how are you left feeling?

Of course it is insufficient to merely answer questions. Specific points will require further explanation; a real problem is more than just an idea needing interrogation and investigation. It represents a threat to the helpee's ability to satisfy 'felt need' in a genuine and satisfying way. By addressing the relevant questions the helper and the helpee will be able to be more precise about the nature and scale of the problem. This in turn will also give a deeper understanding of the broader issues surrounding the problem.

Leigh (1983) provides a good summary of the Kepner-Tragoe method. This method provides additional questions and direction which is likely to assist in the problem diagnosis stage. These questions will include:

☐　　What is distinctive about the actual problem?

☐　　To whom, or what, is the problem attached?

☐　　Where is the problem?

☐　　Where isn't the problem?

☐　　What is different about this particular problem?

☐　　What's different about, or what's changed, in the period the problem occurred?

☐　　How big is the problem?

☐　　Is the problem getting bigger or smaller?

☐　　What is distinctive about the size or growth of the problem?

At the conclusion of the problem-diagnosis stage the helper should be clearer about what needs to be undertaken next, and during the process through the utilisation of specific skills (which will be discussed later in this chapter) the helper will have assisted the helpee in summarising and synthesising his thoughts in reconciling seeming contradictions through the promotion of clear reasoning.

Besides gaining answers to the questions below by encouraging within the helpee genuine self disclosure, further information may also have been obtained:

☐   Is the problem internal or external to the helper?

☐   Is it to do with others?

☐   What are the facts?

☐   What are the opinions?

☐   What are the implications for others?

☐   What are the implications for the helper?

☐   Is it a 'real' problem or a symptom of something else?

☐   What is the time scale, if any, for solution generation?

☐   What other information may be available to assist in solution generation?

☐   Are other professional views required?

The sum of the issue is becoming substantially more precise; more detailed information may still be essential and further analysis and investigation required. For example, a medical examination may be necessary. Stage one of the process must improve understanding of the factors surrounding any problem, and the emphasis at this stage is not upon what any particular solution might be, but on establishing clarification about the nature of the problem. Work at the problem-diagnosis stage is summarised as follows:

☐ clarification of the actual nature of the problem

☐ gathering information or evidence relating to the nature of the problem, and

☐ clarifying what information or evidence may be required in order to further understand the problem

Solution Generation:

Having systematically considered as much evidence as is possible regarding problem diagnosis the solution generation stage is concerned primarily with two issues:

☐ How can solutions be generated?

☐ Which solution should be chosen?

Together the helpee and the helper are likely to be able to devise a large number of solutions and quickly separate the good ones from the poor ones. **Obviously, for a solution to be effective in its implementation it has to be owned by the helpee.**

The philosophical principles (above) acknowledge that the helpee is capable of participating in his own programme of change and that on some level he does know what he needs to do to resolve specific problems.

Actions which make for effective solution generation include flexibility, originality, and critical analysis in order to prevent the helpee from accepting and being satisfied with less-than-meaningful solutions. Therefore, a solution which has stood the test of critical and realistic validation against other options is of course more likely to be successful. Any solution/s must address the following:

Will this course of action get me where I wish to go, and achieve my objectives?

☐ How acceptable/unacceptable is this course of action to me?

☐   Can I live with this course of action?

A widely used technique for generating solutions is that of 'brain-storming'. The ground rules are simple and it is the helper's responsibility to ensure that the helpee keeps to solution generation and does not wander into unrelated arrears. The rules of brain-storming are as follows:

☐   suspend judgement – do not allow criticism of the ideas being generated

☐   let yourself go – encourage wild ideas; it is easier to cut suggestions down to size that to expand them

☐   aim for quantity – encourage as many ideas as possible. This increases the possibility of finding a useful solution

☐   add to the ideas already stated encourage without criticism new possibilities for the ones received, and

☐   clarify ideas already received – when a solution is clarified it can often be expanded

Egan (1980) is a good reference for a more complete discussion on the brain-storming technique. The helper and the helpee exploring solutions and brain-storming, at its best, reduces the probability of making premature choices. The results of brain-storming are rough and ready but can quickly generate many solutions. Moreover, the results can act as an agenda for further evaluation of the problem.

Once the brain-storming exercise has been completed, the contents can be sorted into related groupings from which the generation of solutions can be planned. Potential solutions can then be reviewed against the defined problem in order to assess viability. The helper and the helpee will now be clear about potential solutions, and other solutions which may require further investigations.

A priority checklist of options can be drawn up by placing a weighting on each one in terms of its particular appropriateness in relation to chosen outcomes. In addition, further criteria against which the range of solutions may be compared are as follows:

- ☐ Is the time scale for implementation of the solution reasonable?

- ☐ Will the solution be supported by others affected by the problem?

- ☐ Has the helpee all the resources necessary to support the implementation of the solution?

- ☐ In what ways may the solution fail?

- ☐ Who may wish the solution to fail?

The goal at the solution generation stage is, after all, to estimate the best solution (and adjust if necessary) to reduce the possibility of adverse outcomes, and to increase the probability of positive results arising as a consequence of solution implementation.

For the solutions to be effective they must possess the power to resolve problems and be acceptable to the helpee who actually has the responsibility of implementing the solution. Action at the solution-generation stage is summarised as follows:

- ☐ What alternative options are there?

- ☐ What are the pros and cons of the given alternatives?

- ☐ What is the order of priority of selected solutions?

- ☐ What are the implications for each solution?

Problem solving often entails various degrees of trial and error and, as already indicated, may involve going back in order to refine the problem, and reconsider a range of factors before finally agreeing upon a given solution.

Implementation of Solution:

The essential feature at this stage is reflected in the adage 'actions speak louder than words'. The diagnostic stage clearly emphasizes a rational orientation to understanding the nature of the problem. The solution-generation stage emphasizes the creation of ideas which will then be weighed against various criteria. The implementation stage is the Cinderella of the problem-solving process. It is impossible to implement a solution and not have certain factors change as a result. Certain previous behaviours or activities will discontinue and new behaviours and activities will begin. Things will be different! The implementation stage involves the helpee in questions like:

- What am I to do?

- When am I to do it?

- How am I going to do it?

Putting the solution into effect is the vital test of the helping process. The ability of the helper to extend the processes in problem solving to other situations is the real test of his understanding and is also the basis of progress. Any implementation plan will assist in focusing on the solution and ensure, as far as is possible, that the helpee is working on the agreed plan of action. An implementation plan will define action, and this can be written down and agreed:

- define what behaviour/s or task/s will now be undertaken, and how will these be integrated into a more meaningful experience for the helpee.

- define what specific time each day, if appropriate, will the above be initiated

- define how the above will be implemented to relation to other people, again if appropriate

- defining what resources, for example, financial, will be necessary for successful implementation

113

☐ define where the above will be taking place in terms of, if appropriate, location

☐ define who else may be involved, as appropriate, in the implementation process so that they know why a particular course of action is being pursued, so they may also be accountable for, and know, to what the extent is their own accountability

Implementation plans enable the helper to assist the helpee in keeping the implementation strategy on course. With such detailed planning and consideration regarding implementation of solutions then, potentially, better outcomes become a realistic expectation.

An implementation plan allows all parties to become aware of what progress is being made and what adjustments, if any, need also to be made. Plans which are specified and widely agreed will give a sense of purpose and direction to the solution, and these will be reflected in statements like:

☐ I/We know what we are trying to do

☐ I/We know when we have achieved it

The interrelationship of all of the elements needs to be made clear and understood as these are not separate elements in themselves but part of a whole. Work at the implementation stage is summarised as follows:

☐ what I (and possibly others) am to do

☐ when it is to be done

☐ what implementation plans will be followed, and

☐ how will I know if I am successful?

Review:

The problem-solving process involves movement through the stages of problem diagnosis, solution generation, implementation and review. The review stage clearly examines the successes or otherwise of the implementation of the solution and the appropriateness of the solution. The review stage examines the implementation plan against the following:

☐ Has the plan been effective in achieving its aim?

☐ What parts were more successful than others?

☐ What parts, if any, require adjustment?

☐ What parts, if any, require development and further consideration?

☐ What parts, if any, require further definition?

☐ To what extent does the helpee remain committed and motivated to the solution?

☐ What elements of the solution have been overlooked?

☐ How does the helpee think and feel now about the solution and its relation to the problem?

☐ How do significant others think and feel about the solutions?

Finally, is it still the 'right' solution?

Solutions are sometimes ineffective, not because they are poorly implemented but because they are inappropriate. The solution may be based upon adequate understanding of the problem but inadequate to its resolution. **Every solution incorporates within it a theory of what is the problem and if the solution fails, it may be the underlying theory that is at fault rather than the solution or its execution.** If the solution is based upon faulty information the chances of error are clearly increased, hence the need for consistent monitoring and analysis at the implementation stage.

Other learned habits may get in the way of effective problem solving and such factors, for example, bias or prejudice, or reluctance and poor motivation, are likely to interfere with the implementation and are therefore necessarily explored during the review stage. Moreover, erroneous rationalisation of one particular element within the implementation plan, by making it unacceptable, may destroy the whole plan, hence the dynamic nature of the four-stage model.

Transactional Analysis and Problem Solving:

Throughout the problem-solving process, the helper is facilitating the helpee to identify the problem, checking accuracy and reconciling seeming contradictions and placing the problem in perspective with regard to all the multifaceted influences in the helpee's life. In TA this process, and the reasoning involved, explores all the ego states.

To begin, the helpee would be asked to activate his Adult ego state. That is, looking rationally and objectively, and using that ego state to progress through the following steps. Clearly, some steps may not apply to all problems. By using the Adult ego state the helpee will be asked to:

- define the problem and write it down – he may find that what he thought was the basic problem is not the basic problem

- the helpee would then be asked to explore from his parent ego state – both nurturing and critical – opinions, information, and behaviour concerning the problem

- he will list from his own Parent ego state what each of his own parents might say or do about the problem,

- he will listen to his parents speaking in his head and write down their 'shoulds', and 'oughts' and so on and would be asked, again from his Parent ego sate what he believed they

116

avoided saying, and also what their non-verbal messages may be

☐ next, the helpee will be asked to consider his Child ego state. Remember, needs, wants and feelings are derived from the Child ego state

☐ the helpee will be asked to list the feelings he has in relation to the problem and will be asked to investigate whether the feelings are 'legitimate' or learned and adapted responses

☐ he will be asked to consider whether or not any psychological games are being played in connection with the problem, and

☐ he will be asked to consider whether the problem fits into his constructive, destructive, or non-productive Script. Also he would be asked to indicate whether any manipulative roles are being played by him, for example, Persecutor, Rescuer, or Victim

At this stage the helpee will be requested to evaluate the above information received from his own Parent and Child ego states with his Adult ego state in terms of:

☐ What Parent ego state attitudes hinder you in solving the problem?

☐ What Parent ego state attitudes aid you in solving the problem?

☐ What Child ego state feelings and adaptations hinder you in solving the problem?

☐ What Child ego state feelings and adaptations aid you in solving the problem?

☐ What solution would please your Parent ego state? Would it be appropriate or destructive for you to do this? And, what solution would please your Child ego state? Would it be appropriate or destructive?

117

The helpee would then be asked to imagine alternative ways to solve the problem and would be asked to be as creative and intuitive as possible so as to come up with as many possibilities as he can.

Once possibilities have been generated the helpee will be asked to consider what internal and external resources are available, appropriate, or required to meet each suggested solution. The helpee would be asked to, estimate the **probability of success** for each of the alternatives and eliminate those that are impractical or unsuitable.

Two or three of the most suitable solutions would be selected on the basis of the facts clarified in terms of the nature of the problem, and the helpee will be asked to identify which option he believes is the most viable concerning the resolution of the problem. The helpee will then be asked to **consider very carefully the effects of his decision**: decisions that make you 'feel good' may be satisfying to all ego states. A decision that makes you feel uncomfortable may have your Parent and/or Child ego states fighting against it. This may actually be harmful to yourself or others – or may simply be the wrong option. The helpee would then be asked:

☐ to establish the contract and arrangements necessary for the implementation of the decision and he will use his Adult ego state to raise all appropriate questions concerning any contract or arrangements, and

☐ the option will then be implemented. If possible, it is useful to test the chosen option in a small way before full implementation

Following implementation the helpee will be asked to evaluate the strengths and weaknesses of the plan of action as it progresses, and consider making adjustments as necessary.

Most importantly, the helpee will be given 'permission' to enjoy his success and not to be overly cast down by his failure.

Often, out of eagerness and good intentions, the helper must remain aware of the potential for he himself acting in a symbiotic way at the implementation stage and wishing to 'help' the helpee, this simply deprives the helpee of the opportunity to do any real problem solving for himself. **It must be remembered that the role of the helper is that of fostering independence with the helpee.**

Further Comment:

In enabling the helpee to develop efficiency in defining and clarifying problems, the helper will regularly be asking the helpee 'What do you think?' In specific terms this means:

☐ Is your thinking in terms of you decision regarding the problem based on assumption of reality?

☐ Are you being completely honest with yourself concerning the agreed action?

☐ Is your thinking telling you that you are happy about the goals you now wish to achieve and are you sure you wish to expend time and energy on goal-related activities?

☐ Do you think you fully understand the implications of the goals you are now setting yourself?

☐ Is your thinking clear concerning ways in which you will be evaluating your own progress?

☐ Do you think your feelings are happy with the responses you have given me?

The helper will be aiming to keep the helpee's attention fully focused on the agreed goals and try, in conjunction with the helpee, to eliminate anything which interferes with the achievement of those goals. In summary, the helpee will know:

☐ what he is trying to change

☐ how that change will be achieved, and

☐   when it has been achieved

The helpee will also have gained insight into:

☐   why he thinks, feels, and behaves in the way he does

☐   why he thinks, feels, and behaves differently in different situations

☐   what self-learning is necessary to remedy his destructive thinking, feeling, and behaving

☐   what his thinking, feeling, and behaving might be expressing in terms of meeting needs, and

☐   how his needs might be met in more satisfying ways

How can A Practitioner Evaluate His Work?

There are various approaches to evaluating the quality of work undertaken by the helper, the maintenance of standards being central considerations. A helper can:

☐   look at the entire process with given individual clients. He can select particular points on the process, for example the solution-generation stage in the model

☐   the quality of his interaction with the helpee

☐   he can work, in conjunction with the helpee, and review process and ask for feedback, and

☐   he can ask for supervision from a neutral party

Self-evaluation for the effective helper is an integral aspect of the total helping process. This ongoing evaluation provides the information upon which the helper's further development and acquisition of skill can be planned and guided. Of course, underlying any meaningful self-evaluation must be the helper's own motivation to enrich and promote his abilities.

CHAPTER SEVEN

Contracts and the Management of Time

Helping others is contractual. This means that the helpee is responsible with the helper for determining his own treatment goals and is an active participant in the process.

A contract is an agreement between the helper and the helpee which outlines the goals, stages, and conditions of the helping relationship. The contract makes those intentions explicit. The contract will confirm the number, times, duration, and venue, and include a progress-review point, for example, after six sessions an assessment of progress will take place.

The part of the contract associated with the helpee's expectations will follow from the initial helping sessions. The contract should be brief and stated in words which are clearly understandable to the helpee. It should also be as 'behaviourally' specific as possible so that its attainment can be readily ascertained – certainly by the helpee and preferably by outside sources. **An acceptable helping contract is any desired change in which the helpee ends up feeling progress has been made.** Any specific behavioural change issues should be written in a positive way so as not to subtly reinforce old behaviours. For example, if the assessed problem for the helpee is 'anger' the contract might be written 'to behave in ways that are personally more satisfying', there is no mention of anger.

The initial assessment clarifies the problem enabling the contract to be drawn and using the above as an example, 'anger', the contract will be defined in terms of completing a goal rather than refining a goal. Here are some examples of contract:

☐   to think and feel and react appropriately

☐   to get my needs met in honest ways

☐   to work on looking competent, and

☐   I will express my feelings appropriately and behave in non-threatening ways

In other words, the assessment attempts to establish what model of the world the helpee has (related to be a specific problem) and the contract summarizes the position the helpee wishes to get to in positive terms. By following this approach, what may appear to be insurmountable problems or obstacles for the helpee can be reduced to something definite and which the helpee can cope and feel comfortable with. The following simplified process provides an example:

Helpee: "I'm angry".

Helper: "With what?"

Helpee: "With people".

Helper: "What is it about people that makes you angry?"

Helpee: "I can't trust people."

Helper: "What is it that stops you from trusting people?" or, "What would happen if you trusted people?" or, "Can you trust some people?"

A suitable contract may then be: 'form relationships with your neighbours and learn to trust them.'

Change means doing things differently and if we are doing things differently it means that the way in which we manage our time will be different. If being 'angry' meant, for example, the helpee spent much of his time sitting alone in a bar and drinking alcohol, then as he gives up old behaviours and replaces them with new ones he has also to decide how he will manage his time differently. Time management must be considered as part of the implementation-of-change strategy.

The Management of Time:

Human beings are, in the main, naturally gregarious beings. We are alive, we are dynamic, and always move towards our own comforts. By this it is meant we do things that are 'satisfying' in terms of meeting needs, for example, being with others, exploring interests and even, for some people, committing suicide.

The growing and developing individual structures or manages their time effectively, and in a way which is meaningful to them. Many people in difficulty with themselves endeavour to cope with the difficulties by pulling away, by isolating themselves, by not involving themselves, 'What can I do', 'I'm bored', 'I just sit and look into space'.

The particular ways in which a person structures his time depends upon whether or not he feels positive about himself and others, and reflects the kinds of strokes or patterns of recognition he is seeking to give and receive.

There are six ways of managing time, and at any given moment each of us is involved in one or more of these time structures.

Withdrawal:

People withdraw from others either by removing themselves physically or by removing themselves psychologically. Withdrawal behaviour is reflected in statements, like, 'I need to be alone', 'When things are difficult I go for a walk'.

Withdrawal mechanisms are likely it to be adaptations out of the necessity for self-protection from pain or conflict. Withdrawal is usually safe, requiring little emotional investment, but does not provide stroking or recognition from others.

A certain amount of withdrawal is healthy and normal behaviour. Everyone needs to collect their thoughts. Of course, some people avoid withdrawal because they are afraid to be alone and choose, instead, to structure time in ways which distracts them from their personal thoughts and feelings. On the other hand, if people spend too much time withdrawing they become lonely, deprived of strokes, and depressed.

It has been said that the ability to be alone, to feel safe when alone, only comes from experience of being close to another. Often, being alone for some people is likely to be a very disturbing experience similar to, 'unfocused depression' or a state of 'mourning' resulting from the loss of psychological unity.

Depression and anxiety indicate conflict, and withdrawal, paradoxically, is likely to be a first move towards a search for help as the act of withdrawing may be the first 'admission' of a problem. Anxiety consists in part of the feeling of helplessness in the face of a 'hostile' words, and leads to the development of more 'neurotic' defences, like withdrawal, and unhealthy strategies for coping with the world. If there is no one to turn to, or for whatever reason the individual feels unable to turn to others, he may develop the neurotic need to withdraw.

Rituals:

Rituals are stereotyped series of transactions that are highly predictable. The most common rituals of any culture are those of greeting, 'Good morning, how are you?'

If a whole life is primarily patterned on ritualistic living, growth and development are inhibited, because they do not risk new creative ways of thinking, feeling, and behaving. Although rituals do provide some superficial contact with others the emotional yield is low. A person who structures his time primarily in withdrawal and rituals, is likely to experience deprivation and loneliness. Customary hellos, goodbyes, and hugs may be, in proportion, positive anchors, but obviously contain major limitations. The person who is stuck in rituals and wishes to move into more intense interpersonal exchanges may need to progress slowly, similarly the person who is withdrawn.

Pastimes:

Pastiming often follows a ritualistic greeting. When people are pastiming they simply talk to one another about subjects that are of little consequence: the weather, cars, football results, and TV programmes are examples.

The psychological game, 'Ain't It Awful' is another common pastime, without any suggestion of what could be undertaken to make matters better, except talking! Pastiming can give us a needed break and a chance to relax. Pastiming provides people with the opportunity of becoming acquainted and perhaps leads them into a deeper relationship. If, however, pastiming is carried to excess an overwhelming amount of time may be taken away from other forms of time-management which are not, as yet, fully part of the individual's time management repertoire.

Activities:

Work, hobbies, and chores are activities. Activities produce strokes in many ways. When a job is well done, positive strokes are often obtained in the form of praise from friends or work colleagues. Of course, negative strokes may be received if a person does a job poorly, or is working with people who find fault easily. Strokes may be intrinsic rather the extrinsic – when we are able to see the fruits of our own efforts and feel good about it. The process of helping is essentially an activity, since its purpose is goal orientated. It is the responsibility of the helper to ensure that whatever activities the helper, and the helpee are helpee may be involved in, these activities are designed and aimed towards the desired outcome and treatment goals.

Psychological Games:

Psychological Games, as already suggested in an earlier chapter, tend to be an unproductive use of time since they are played to avoid anything else, for example: like solving a problem, making a decision, getting close to people, or involvement in meaningful activity. Moreover, games can be extremely destructive for one or both players, 'that's a good piece of work you finished, ...considering!'.

Intimacy:

Intimacy strokes go much deeper that ritual, pastime, or activity strokes. Intimacy strokes are the kind we give and receive from open relationships with no ulterior transactional motive. During moments of intimacy people do not try to get anything out of each other. They are not possessive or demanding. They are simply being with one another, listening to one another, and caring about one another. At such times people feel appreciative, tender, and affectionate. For many people intimacy may be uncomfortable. They may be fearful and distrustful of others, choose to keep their distance, and avoid closeness. They unknowingly choose games, rituals, or pastime as a way of avoiding being real, or too emotionally close to other people. This is not to say that such people do not wish to experience more intimacy in their lives, but for them to accomplish such is for whatever reason or problem, not easy. The helper will use positive stroking language as a beginning in the process of enabling the helpee to receive, and experience, positive strokes.

Maintaining eye contact (in a non-threatening way) may also enhance closeness. Exchanges involving, 'I and/or you' and involving the sharing of feelings, and staying in the 'here and now', are other techniques.

The helping environment must be conducive to trust, risk, and change. Generally before people can experience intimacy they must work through their personal fears and blocks about intimacy, and be willing to risk fully experiencing their natural feelings and meeting their needs in a genuine way. A person who believes that he and others are OK will risk being open and intimate in many more circumstances than will the person who doubts his or others, OKness.

It is the helper's example in the helping situation that contains an important part of the helping, and change process. His example influences attitude, behaviour, motivation, and the development of the helping relationship. How he listens, attends, and engages his whole self in helping underlies all of the discussion, and techniques referred throughout this book. In short, the interpersonal dimension is the most critical element within the helping relationship.

CHAPTER EIGHT

<u>Being with the Helpee</u>

We have discussed methods, techniques, process, process of change, and so on within the realm of problem solving and becoming. We know what we are trying to achieve. The helper provides the helpee with the experience of being understood. Being effective, particularly in the early stages of the helping-relationship, the helper gives his full attention, consideration, and energy to the helpee. Thus, doing his utmost to understand what the helpee is really saying. The helpee then becomes more fully engaged in the process of his own self-discovery and self-understanding. The helper listens and gives his full attention to the helpee. For example:

Helpee: "I don't see how this is going to get me anywhere"

Helper: "I hear you saying that trying to work things out is difficult for you"

Helpee: "It's alright for you"

Helper: "What about you – I'd like to spend some time getting to know you better and then may be I'll be more able to be helpful?"

Helpee: "No one knows who I really am and how I really feel"

Helpee: "It gets you down because you are not seen for who you really are".

The helper is endeavouring to show empathy, and understanding, and is responding in a way which encourages the helpee to continue to self disclose. Empathy is like placing yourself in the other's shoes – to see the world through the other person's eyes. To feel the things the helpee feels and to experience the world from his point of view. By showing empathy, the helper not only places himself 'in the skin' of the helpee but is also able to demonstrate through the language and responses that he is in the helpee's 'skin' and is communicating that back to the helpee. This skill also provides a mirror for the helpee to hear and see himself as he really is. This can only be achieved by listening and attending fully to the helpee, and will also communicate to the helpee that he is being cared for, and that there is a belief in his ability to do something about his problem and his life.

By fully listening and then responding the helper will 'direct' the helpee into being more specific and concrete about his feelings and experiences. In discussing 'grandiosity' it was shown how words like 'always', 'never' need to be challenged and made specific in order to enable the helper to understand fully what is being said and what the helpee is experiencing.

The helper is endeavouring to put together a picture of the helpee, to give direction to the process, and is attempting to get the helpee to see and understand himself at a deeper level, this demands of the helper, genuineness. That is, the helper being as real as he can be, bearing in mind the helper is still there to help the other person. So, if the helper has feelings and thoughts about the helpee it would be more helpful for him to ask of himself where these feelings are coming from rather than place them on the helpee.

If the helper is being genuine he will be able to confront the helpee with regard to 'saying things that are normally left unsaid', or reflecting back what is being observed. For example:

Helpee: "I feel really relaxed now" (said when the helpee is agitated and drumming his fingers).

Helper: "this is not what I see, your body language is telling me you are not relaxed".

The insights gained from listening, attending, mirroring back, being concrete, and showing empathy will create new insights for the helpee which, in conjunction with an agreed course of action associated with a given problem or problems will hopefully be integrated by the helpee as part of his own development.

Much material for potential use in 'being with the helpee' is lost. Almost any exchange contains within it the potential for exploration. The helper, with experience and practice, will be using his own intuition in deciding which statements require further exploration. **(See Handout Nine: Considering My Script and Other Questions)** For example:

- Which family members does the helper get along with best, may give some indication of the kind or relationships, and the nature of preferred relationships, for example, 'I prefer being with my grandfather as he doesn't criticise me all the time'

- What were your parent's favourite sayings about life? For example, they may have been, 'you can't trust people', or 'don't show your feelings'

The helper in 'being with' the helpee is getting to know what values and view of 'self' the helpee has accumulated from his experiences.

Some people will find it more difficult than others to discuss thoughts and feelings. (**Handout Ten: Exploring Thoughts and Feelings, and Handout Eleven: Further Exploration of Self)** will, as with the majority of the Handouts, help with self-disclosure.

Introjection and Projection:

We encounter the outer world, its impact, the situations we live through, and the people we meet, not only as external experiences but also by taking them into the self they then become part of our inner life. 'Being with the helpee' shows the helper how the helpee may shift from being simply himself towards being more like what he thinks is expected of him. This shift away from being himself involves a partial identification with parents, significant others (including the helper), and the internalisation of their attitudes, thus influencing their helpee's reaction to external events. This process Freud described as introjection, in other words, characteristics and attitudes belonging to others which one attributes to oneself.

Projection is a phenomenon in which characteristics belonging to oneself are attributed to others. Introjection, as already postulated, indicates an attempt on the part of us to model ourselves upon those we either have to please, or those who please us. At the same time, we come to regard aspects of ourselves as unpleasant and so deny them. These unpleasant characteristics will be attributed or projected to others and we are condemning in them that which we cannot accept in ourselves. For example, the selfish person sees selfishness in others and condemns others for being selfish.

Introjection and projection, although they are rooted in infancy, are not exclusively infantile processes. This interaction continues throughout life, becoming modified in the course of maturation. Moreover, introjection and projection never lose their importance in how we relate to the world around us. These processes help to mould our impression of our surroundings, often in fantasy, and by introjection our picture of the external world changes and will influence what goes on in our minds. Thus, an inner world is built up which is partly a reflection of our perceived external world. (Klein, 1963).

It follows that, as a result of the experiences an individual undergoes in relation to the various components of his environment, his self-concept and world view emerges. The reactions of significant adults, especially in a child's world, are of crucial importance. By constantly nagging and failing him, adults succeed in convincing him that he is stupid and worthless, and leads him to confirm that viewpoint by his behaviour.

Ronald Laing's theories in parental programming appear strikingly similar to the concepts of introjection, projection, and life positions, as the emphasis is upon environmental responses (strokes), feelings of security, self esteem, and inferiority – the 'OK and the not OK' postures.

For example, Laing argues that the most potent parental injunctions come in 'is'. Through the parent telling the child what he 'is', the parent is implying an expected adaptive response about what to 'be' and what to 'do' and 'not do'. The attribution is made by the child's parent, but the injunction itself is an internal operation carried out by the child.

A 'don't think' injunction, for example, is derived from a child being told he is 'stupid'. Moreover, Laing in, 'The Politics of the Family', states that the 'key for communication of this kind is probably non-verbal language'. This parallels the TA view that injunctions are largely communicated non-verbally by conveying 'psychological' messages.

Non-verbal Communication:

Through our dress, body language, and posture, we convey many messages in order to either engage people or avoid them. People whose shoulders droop, who whine, and look anxious, may be conveying a message which is saying, 'poor me I need taking care of'. Alternatively, a person scowling at the world may be conveying a message, 'keep away from me'. The kind of clothing we wear, and the non-verbal gestures we use may be giving out, for example, messages like, 'I'm available' or 'I don't care'. These messages are often part of a life-script pattern but beneath them usually there is a second message like, for example, 'I'm not really as helpless as I look', 'I do really wish to be close to people, I'm not really available'.

Psychological Drivers:

The essence of these often negative, restrictive and double messages is, contained, in the concept of **Drivers**, these **are life-script directives** (Woollams and Brown, 1979). Drivers contain socially acceptable moral judgements and value statements, which please significant others. However, since it is not possible for the individual to respond to these messages all the time, they are destructive in the long run, although they do lead to script decisions. These script directives have been divided into five groupings:

☐ be perfect

☐ hurry up

- try hard

- please me, and

- be strong

These attributions, are the product of consistent reinforcing actions from parents onto the child, they do however contain a second side! For example, a boy who is taught to emphasise toughness may also be internalising, 'don't show my feelings'. A girl who is learning that looking good for others is a way of getting strokes may be internalising, 'I have to please other people and must not leave them'.

Therefore, there are **two sides to Drivers,** although of course, they are two sides of the same coin. They may look different but they are intimately inter-related and are in basic agreement. The two sides are as follows:

- be perfect – but fail

- hurry up – grow up quickly/don't be a child

- try hard – but don't make it

- please me – don't please yourself, and

- be strong – don't feel

The helper, by being with and attending to the helpee will, through the quality of the interpersonal interactive process, be giving the helpee 'permission' to be himself, and to be genuine. The basic permissions implied are explicit in the process:

- you have a right to be your own judge;

- you have a right to change your mind;

- you have a right not to justify your behaviour to others;

☐   you have a right to make mistakes and be responsible for the consequences;

☐   you have a right to say, 'I don't know'

☐   you have a right to say, 'I don't understand', and

☐   you have a right to say, 'I don't care'

It is Ok to succeed, it is OK to feel, it is OK to be happy.

Rethinking Failures:

The helpee will have 'failures' – these are inevitable. No system of helping has universal validity or absolute success. It is likely that the study of failures could help the helper improve his methods more meaningfully than just examining his successes! So, what is to be 'done' about failures? We have discussed earlier the need for the helper to be consistently evaluating his own skills and abilities, **so how should the helper respond to failure?**

Firstly, it is suggested, the helper may need to go back and questions the initial contract. For example, a person may be contracted to 'deal with aggressive feelings more appropriately' but really needed to be working on 'getting close to people'. The helpee's resistance to change could be the result of a failure to identify what he really needed.

Another problem may have been to do with the helpee's projection of issues. That is, the helpee generalising his world view or script decision into the helping relationship. For example, the over-complying helpee who may have been scripted to always 'be nice to people', and deny his own needs. Consequently, he is pleasant to the helper but fails to improve emotionally or working on problems.

Again, as stated earlier, people are sometimes slow to change because change means 'giving up' familiar and certain forms of behaviour. They really know that something is wrong with their lives but may go on defending in the belief that defending is equal to functioning.

The lesson for the helper is, as a priority, to look for the feeling that is supporting the behaviour, or thought, and the behaviour that is supporting a feeling. One way to achieve this is to quietly and caringly intensify confrontation and hence the helpee will increase or exaggerate his behaviour. Nevertheless, the helpee may continue to discount information regarding problems, change possibilities, and ways of taking care of himself. **Change will not result until the helpee also realises that change is possible.** Inevitably there are occasions when this stage will never be reached.

Change means meeting crises or problems in new ways. **Becoming does not mean becoming free of pain or distress. It means learning to face such realities differently,** to change that way we interact with others, and most importantly, to learn to tolerate anxiety or uncertainty.

The process of change is frightening, but the greatest fear is change itself. New behaviour is unknown, threatening, and risky. New strains must be handled, endured and coped with in the process of growth. There is always the danger of some regression, or of giving up. The helpee may meet an old situation in which his hostility will again flare up, and he finds himself in his old reaction pattern. This is why continuing support may need to be built into any subsequent contract. It must be remembered, that the **two major components underpinning the helping process argued for here are:**

☐ that the helpee knows cognitively and viscerally what he needs to do to get 'well', and

☐ and, that he can take responsibility for functioning differently

Termination of the Helping Relationship:

The question of termination of helping is often a difficult one to answer. No helpee reaches perfection and there will always be issues to work through and ways in which to improve. At some stage, however, the helping relationship reaches a point of diminishing returns. The time, energy, and possibly money, spent in helping outweigh the benefits which a given helpee is receiving.

The final decision about concluding helping will involve the helper and the helpee. The helper's responsibility is to give feedback regarding how he sees the helpee doing, especially with regard to the change goals as defined within the contract. Has the helpee met the goals as outlined in the contract, if not why not and, is terminating helping a way the helpee is using to avoid the contract?

The helper will need to hear from the helpee how he is feeling and thinking about termination:

☐   Does termination make sense to him?

☐   Does he feel satisfied with the present ways of taking care of himself?

☐   Is he providing for himself adequate nurturing, and protection, for continued growth?

At other times, the termination will be initiated directly by the helper. When this occurs the reason should be very clear. It may be that the helpee is so involved with his own destructive and distorted behaviours that these are interfering so significantly with the helping process that they completely obstruct any opportunity for progress. These are difficult decisions. But the helper must be honest with himself – there will always be people for whom, for various reasons, it is impossible to work with, and this must be acknowledged.

Conclusion:

The methods and experiences described indicate that when an individual confronts his thoughts, feelings, and behaviour, he comes into contact with likely explanations as to why he feels, thinks, and behaves as he does. By acting upon this information in a supportive, reactive, attentive, and 'confrontative' helping relationship with a skilled helper, increased awareness can lead to a transformative experience for the helpee, which results in purposeful change in his world view.

The helping process allows the individual to experience all states of consciousness, and through the experience of the helping process gain a world view which incorporates co-operation and caring. He re-examines and revises the world view that may have reinforced or created personal problems and disharmony. This re-examination leads to the development of a self which is viable and life enhancing.

All helping or therapeutic approaches can be used as instruments of conformity, domination or liberation – it is the helper and his skill which ensures helping is a therapeutic and liberating experience.

An effective helper will be directly involved in his own self-actualizing potential which, in turn, means that the **helping experience for others will be active around: problem solving, care of feelings, care of oneself, and care of others.**

CHAPTER NINE

Response—Ability

This chapter tries to encapsulate and embrace the spirit of this book, so let us conclude by listening to a self-actualizing person:

"...I have no need for a false self-image to try to 'tell' me what I am like, or what I should think, should do, or should feel. Any image I have of myself is a fantasy, an idea, if based upon a false self-image. I become a person who identifies with an idea of myself instead of with the reality of my true feelings, experiences and behaviour. I become split between what I think I am, and what I am.

My false self-image tells me to chase and seek goals which feed that false self-image. I then become frightened if I fail to achieve those goals. Of course, the goals I seek are to impress you. I try to convince you, and me, that I am my false image. The more I try to impress you the more I fear your bad opinion of me. My fears grow upon each other and take me further from the actual reality of me. I become a shadow of my true self. I eventually become angry or withdrawn, feel worthless, and, of course, finally become unwell.

I, like you, makes decisions from the standpoint of – how can I best get along in the world? Unfortunately, these decisions are often inappropriate, or over-generalized to inappropriate times, places, or people. My false self-image developed from compliances with your expectations of me – with what I imagined you expectations to be of me. I become what you expected of me. I become a response to what you said I am. My false self-image may have appeared to have made me feel good but in fact, I felt bad.

As new experiences follow, I tend more and more to evaluate new situations in the light of the previous generalizations and experiences. If I try harder to maintain my false self-image then my decisions about, how can I best get along in the world, become harder to make?

I wish to gain contact with my actual experience and my real responses. I wish to connect the fragments of me. I wish to live in a flexible and flowing way with the events that fill my life so that I have no need for a false self-image. I want to be in touch with my actual experiences of the world. To be balanced and centred in my sensing and responding to the world. I don't wish to act differently to how I feel. I don't wish to reduce my contact with what I am actually experiencing. I have no need for a false self-image.

I know that a full awareness of my experience requires full acceptance of that experience as it is. With a false self-image I actually moved away from my real self. I allowed a falsification of my life by acting differently to the way in which I feel. I developed a false self-image which is not based upon the reality of how I actually feel. I know that to find my real self I have to regain contact with my existence be increasing my awareness. This means that maintaining contact with my existence has to become an integral part of my everyday life.

I have now become through my senses more aware of the outside world – what I see, hear, smell, taste, and touch. More aware of my inner world – how I feel inside my skin, muscular tensions, discomfort, well-being, and emotions and feelings. These two kinds of awareness embrace all that I can know about Now, as I experience Now. The facts of my existence are here within each moment.

By using my mental energies I can discover more about each moment by explaining and interpreting to myself feelings and perceptions and behaviour as they occur.

A helper taught me a technique which has enabled me to increase my self-awareness and begin to resolve the split between myself and a false self, constructed from the demands others placed upon me. You may wish to join me in the exercise. You also probably experience some kind of split or conflict. I used to think that my conflicts were with others, and failed to realise how much of the conflict, and conflicts, actually belong to me and are within me.

Now close your eyes and sit comfortably on a chair or the floor and imagine you are looking at yourself sitting in front of you. Form a picture of yourself sitting there in front of you. How is this image sitting? What is this image of you wearing? What facial expressions do you see? Silently criticise this image of yourself, or, if you choose to, speak aloud.

Tell yourself what you should, and should not do. Make a list of criticisms. Listen to your voice. How does it sound? How do you feel emotionally and physically as you do this? Now, alter places with your image, become this image of yourself, and answer those criticisms. Be aware of what you say in response to these criticisms. What does your tone of voice express? How do you know feel?

Switch roles whenever you wish to, but keep the dialogue going. Be aware of all the details of what is going on in you, as you do this. Does your posture change for each role? Are you physically feeling different? Do you really talk to each other, or do you avoid contact, or frustration? How do you think and feel about this other speaker, and see how this other speaker responds? Do you notice any changes as you continue this dialogue? Now be quiet.

Review in your mind this dialogue, and as you look back is there anything else about the conversation that you notice? Now open your eyes and express what you think happened. You may be saying things like: I found one role more dominant than the other, or one sounded like my mother, or one kept avoiding issues, or one was more joyful, and the other depressed and so on. Whatever occurs in this exercise goes on between different parts of you. If there is conflict in your dialogue this conflict is between parts of yourself. Even if you alienate one part, and call it society or husband or boss, remember if you or I participate in outside conflicts before clearing the conflicts with us, we create more conflict both inside and outside.

By my taking responsibility for my conflicts, and you taking responsibility for yours, by understanding them and learning from them, the result will be increased awareness. As our awareness increases we can begin to make new decisions about ourselves and the factors affecting out lives. As our awareness increases we begin to settle the 'civil war' which is going on inside of us. As a result of increased awareness we discover for whom the messages in this internal dialogue are really intended – or from where they came. The next step is to direct them outwards!

We direct them outwards from an inward awareness, increased awareness gained from an ongoing internal dialogue, will free us from false feelings and behaviour, and move us towards autonomy and genuineness. I discussed with you thoughts on my false self-image and how I found, ultimately, this to be a very destructive feature of my life. I then shared with you a technique, which is essentially about regaining contact with our real self and gaining more self-awareness. As we regain contact with our real self we start to make new decisions about our lives from a position that enhances self-awareness. In other words, we begin to become more genuine.

Genuineness is a behaviour, and is therefore something I can choose or not choose. I can decide to be personally genuine. When I share with others what I genuinely feel, I am showing that I can be trusted. In order to do this I must first be honest with myself. I have to get in touch with my experiencing, and take responsibility for it by expressing it as my experiencing, just like we did in the exercise earlier.

When I respect myself enough to be genuine, others respond with respect. If I put on false behaviour I am hiding my real self. Others may still like me for the image I create, but I am not liked for me. I am in fact manipulating myself to get a certain response from you, a response which holds no real satisfaction because I am not being genuine. When I am being genuine I can receive you fully with the satisfaction of being related with you through me. Relating to you genuinely will not always be joyful. It will sometimes be sad or angry; however, it will always be real and alive.

My increased self-awareness will also make me more aware of you, and open to receive your expression of your awareness, what you are actually saying, or what you might be expressing through your non-verbal behaviour.

Making new decisions about ourselves which move us towards becoming genuine will not be easy. Giving up old behaviours and adopting new behaviours is often frightening because we have become 'secure' with the illusion of who we are.

If you remember, I said a little earlier that we make decisions from the standpoint of – how can I best get along in the world? Our move towards genuineness will involve a shift in what we value. A value shift, in this context, would be, 'I want to be liked for the person I am and will therefore give up false behaviour'. It is very important to say at this stage that this has nothing to do with willpower. Why?

All our behaviours are governed according to values. We all have different dominant values, be they in the area of behaviour, moral conduct, or self-respect. It is possible to change our dominant vales so that we avoid previous conflicts, but this is not willpower. It is simply you or me substituting new values which offer us a higher level of acceptability. The well-behaved individual is said to exercise willpower while the individual who fails to live up to social expectations is said to be lacking in willpower. In fact the difference is related to different dominant values. Change takes place when our values change. The thief and the policeman all have essentially the same needs, but they display different behaviour because they have different values.

So, by establishing genuineness as your dominant value your life will, correspondingly, be more rewarding. You may wish to set aside a period of time each day as silent time when words are only used in emergencies. Use this silent time to take in experiences which would otherwise be lost for words. Be aware of what impulses impel you to speak. If you forget yourself, notice what you say, did you actually communicate, or were your words really useless noise?

Try a silent meal. See how much of the taste and textures of the food you have been losing as a result of meaningless chatter. Silence allows you to become more aware, by becoming more aware you become more genuine.

We all have a great deal of unused potential. Our playing at weakness, or being stupid, is just playing at weakness and being stupid. We are more capable, more intelligent, more able than we believe.

If I become more genuine with myself and insist that others also become more genuine I become immune to manipulations, and at the same time initiate change in them also.

We have to begin this journey of genuineness from where we are. Start here. If I meet you on this journey I trust we will respond to each other with a genuine response-ability..."

Handout One

Client-Centred Helping and Counselling: Summary of Process, the Core Skills, and Principles

Introduction:

The purpose of helping and counselling is to facilitate the alleviation of physical, emotional, psychological, cognitive, and affective distress, and in doing so is focused upon problems of living.

Helping is a process that assists the client in exploring their problems, deciding upon a plan of action, supporting the client through implementation, reviewing progress.

The relationship is non-possessive, emphasizes self-help and choice, uses a repertoire of skills efficiently, with competence, and expertise.

Aims to establish or clarify the nature of concern by: communicating with the client, listening to the client, observing the client, encouraging the client to speak, responding to the client, eliciting clarification and factual information, eliciting emotional information, and recording information.

Involves agreeing with/from the client their chosen course/s of action by establishing with the client the nature of help required, determining the extent and level of help required, and liaising, if necessary, with other professionals with the client's approval and agreement.

In working with the client the helper will use the full range of skills central to the helping-relationship in order to understand, support, and facilitate the client in seeking clarity and options for change.

Maintaining confidentiality, clients need to know that information shared, will be held in confidence, unless the client gives their permission to breach confidentiality. (Exceptions may occur under extreme circumstances when/if the freedom and basic well-being of a third party is threatened)

The helper in discussion with the client will end the relationship as and when appropriate.

Helping and Counselling Skills:

1. Setting-up the process:

    ☐ Introduce yourself, including background experience and qualifications
    ☐ Set time, and explain context, role, and purpose, and
    ☐ Focus on the client's immediate feelings, questions, statements

2. Make responses in the form of statements, feedback, rather than questions.

3. Focus upon the client, their feelings, thoughts, and behaviours, be tentative, focusing on the 'here and now', and try to communicate a sense that promotes the idea 'of working together'.

4. Be aware of cues: verbal, vocal, and non-verbal.

5. Use in particular, the following techniques:

    ☐ **active listening**, is an intention to listen for 'meaning' (not interpretation) involving paraphrasing the client's remarks; paying attention to what and how something is being said; making use of non-verbal cues; confirming with the client what is being received by way of feedback, prompts, seeking clarification.

    ☐ **attending behaviour,** by demonstrating interest and attention to the client by actively attending by giving out messages of welcome, being relaxed, open, showing involvement by appropriately encouraging the client, having good eye contact that is reasonable, non-threatening, having a relaxed and friendly facial expression, making use of physical signs of interest, for example, head nods (this does not mean you are agreeing with what is being said, rather you are interested and encouraging).

☐ **unconditional positive regard,** is when one person is completely accepting towards another person, and is an attitude that is then demonstrated through behaviour.

☐ **being empathic**, is to perceive the internal frame of reference of another with accuracy and meaning which pertain, as if one were the other person, but without losing the as if. This means to sense the hurt and pleasure of another as he senses such and to perceive the causes as he perceives them. If this quality is lost then the state of the helper becomes one of identification. (Note: Sympathy and empathy are similar emotional responses, however, one could feel sympathy without experiencing empathy). Empathy involves making guesses at feelings and causes by going beyond what is explicitly said by the client.

☐ **being congruent,** is when there is a good fit between the real self, the perceived self, end ideal self, thus a consistency with inner feeling and outer display; a congruent person is genuine, real, integrated, transparent. (Training for congruence sounds paradoxical: how can you learn and practice being yourself? Yet one of the aims of the person-centred approach is to help the client to develop greater awareness and acceptance of his own thoughts and feelings. **If it is possible to help the client to become more congruent, then it should be possible for helper to do the same.** The more the helpee can accept himself the more likely it is that he will be able to respond in a personal and genuine way to the client. **Non-congruent people** try to impress, play roles, and hide behind a façade. There are two forms of incongruence: incongruence between the helper's feelings and his awareness of those feelings, and, incongruence between his awareness and the expression of his feelings.

Matters to be Avoided:

☐ **Taking control:** "I want you to talk about this issue today"

☐ **Blaming or assigning responsibility:** "It's all your fault"

☐ **Moralising or saying how you think lives should be led:** "Drinking lots of alcohol is not the most important thing in life"

☐ **Labelling**: "I think you have an inferiority complex"

☐ **Humour and rescuing** (avoids feeling and thinking): "Don't worry about it, you will be alright"

☐ **Non-acceptance of feelings or thoughts:** "You shouldn't be feeling depressed, stop thinking that way"

☐ **Giving Advice**, thus taking 'space' away from the client: "You should stop doing this and do that"

☐ **Interrogating, questioning in threatening ways:** "Explain yourself, when do you do that, why, with who else..."

☐ **Inappropriately talking about yourself:** "You think that is a problem, let me tell you about mine"

☐ **Putting on a façade** (being non-congruent): "I am very experienced in your type of problem"

☐ **Faking, pretending you are interested:** "Yes, that's very interesting" whilst being preoccupied

☐ **Time pressure, looking at the clock**: "Oh, you must be quick I have to go"

The Skilled Helper will watch for:

☐ asking too many questions

☐ using leading questions: "You do like coming to counselling don't you?"

☐ using closed questions: "You do like your father?"

☐ being too probing: "How many relationships have you had?", and

☐ poorly timed questions, for example: asking for an explanation whilst the client is sobbing

Additional Skills are :

☐ use **elaboration:** "Tell me more about that"

☐ seek **clarification and specification:** "Can you say more about that, be more specific?"

☐ elicit **personal reactions**: "How do you think and feel about that?"

☐ use **explanatory hypotheses** in order to help the client to make sense of often conflicting or confusing feelings and motives: "Do you think you feel the way you do because of that?"

☐ use **metaphor** in order to highlight a strong feeling or emotion: "You feel like you are swimming against the tide"

Handout Two

List of Attitudes for Discussion and Development of Own List

1. A general list of attitudes: are these attitudes ones that you hold to be important for yourself, hold for yourself? (www.artmilk.com)

have an open mind
have a sense of humour
be childlike
be environmentally aware
be spiritually aware
act spontaneously
be flexible
practise a non-judgemental attitude
be adventurous
impulsive
curious
honest

know yourself
fun loving
work hard
be socially aware
be creative in everything you do
learn to trust your initiative
be open to change
be patient
be thoughtful
be daring, risk taking
energetic
loving
work on integrity

2. Attitude checklist

General Appearance:	No	Sometimes	Yes
I am happy with my looks			
I am happy with my physical health			
I am happy with my height			
I am happy with my weight			
I am neat in appearance			

Emotional characteristics:	No	Sometimes	Yes
I 'act up' when things do not go my way			
I easily feel 'down'			
I get sulky or angry when I use a game			
I easily feel sorry for myself			
I cry or get angry over small things			
I swear at others or call them names			

Manners:	No	Sometimes	Yes
I am courteous to others			
I am considerate of the feelings of others			
I am courteous to members of my family			
I listen when others are talking and do not interrupt			

Parental relationships:	No	Sometimes	Yes
I talk with my parents			
I listen when my parents talk			
My parents listen to my point of view			

General style of behaviour:	No	Sometimes	Yes
I am shy			
I have a need to seek attention			
I am the 'bossy' type			
I let others push me around			
I daydream when I am supposed to be paying attention			
I enjoy teasing and upsetting others			

Character traits:	No	Sometimes	Yes
I am reliable and follow up on my promises			
I am honest			
I respect the opinions and beliefs of others			
I respect the property of others			
I daydream when I am supposed to be paying attention			
I take the initiative to make new friends			
I expect to be treated with respect by others			
I take responsibility			

Our attitude always influences our choices within the demands of the many and various situations we find ourselves.

Note:

Do you dwell in the past or remain in the present, or future?

Do you only see problems in your situation, or opportunities and learning to also come out of your situation?

Do you feel optimistic towards new experiences or feel pessimistic towards the new?

Are you negative or positive in the midst of problems?

Do you step out with hope and courage, or are you doubtful and discouraged?

Is your cup half-empty or half-full?

Handout Three

A Values List for Discussion and Development of Own List

The following list of values will help you develop a clearer sense of what is most important to you in your life. Mark the values which most resonate with you, and then sort your own list in order of priority. This values list is not exhaustive, it is merely a guide. (www.stevepavlina.com)

acceptance	dependability	justice	self-control
accomplishment	discipline	kindness	sensitivity
acknowledgement	drive	knowledge	service
adaptability	education	leadership	sharing
adventure	efficiency	liberty	sexuality
affection	energy	love	simplicity
affluence	excellence	loyalty	stillness
altruism	experience	making a difference	support
assertiveness	fairness	maturity	teamwork
attractiveness	faith	mindfulness	trust
awareness	fame	modesty	truth
balance	fashion	neatness	unity
beauty	fidelity	obedience	vitality
belonging	fitness	open-mindedness	valour
bliss	flexibility	order	warmth
bravery	freedom	originality	wealth
brilliance	frugality	passion	winning
calmness	fun	peace	wisdom
care	generosity	perfection	youthfulness
celebrity	giving	persistence	zeal
charm	gratitude	philanthropy	
chastity	happiness	piety	
cheerfulness	harmony	playfulness	
closeness	honesty	power	
compassion	humility	privacy	
conformity	humour	prudence	
control	impartiality	reason	
co-operation	industry	relaxation	
courtesy	intelligence	reliability	
curiosity	intimacy	resolve	
decisiveness	intuition	respect	
devotion	joy	sacrifice	

Handout Four

Questions about My Interpersonal Style

How big a part of my life is my interpersonal life?

☐ How much of my day is spent relating to people?

☐ Do I want to spend a lot of time with people, or do I prefer being myself, or am I somewhere in between?

☐ Do I have many friends or few?

☐ Whether many or few, do I usually spend a lot of time with my friends?

☐ Is my life too crowded with people?

☐ Are there too few people in my life? Do I feel lonely much of the time?

☐ Do I prefer smaller gatherings or larger groups? Or do I prefer to be with just one person most of the time?

☐ Do I plan to get together with others, or do I leave getting together to chance – if it happens, it happens?

What do I want, and what do I need, when I spend time with others?

☐ What do I like in other people – that is, what makes me choose them as friends? Is it intelligence or physical attractiveness? Is it the fact that they are good-natured and pleasant or that they have the same values as I do? Do I choose to be with people because they are important or in positions of authority?

☐ Do I choose to be with people who will do what I want to do?

☐ Do I choose to be with people who will take over and make decisions for the two of us?

☐ Do I just spend time with whoever happens to come along?

☐ Are the people I go around with like me or different from me? Or are they in some ways like me and in other ways different? How?

☐ Do I feel that I need my friends more than they need me, or is it the opposite?

☐ Do I let others know what I want from them? Do I let them know directly, or do they find out what in indirect ways?

Do I care about the people in my life?

☐ If I care about others how do I show it?
☐ Do others know I care about them?
☐ Do I take others for granted?
☐ Do I wonder at times whether I care at all?
☐ Do I see myself as being selfish or generous, or in the middle?
☐ Do others see me as self-centred? If so, how?
☐ Do others care for me, how do they show it?

Am I good at relating to people? What are my interpersonal skills like?

☐ Am I good at both understanding others, and letting them know that I understand?
☐ Do I respect others? How well do I communicate that I do respect them?
☐ Am I my real self when I am with others, or do I play games and act phoney at times?
☐ Am I open – that is, willing to talk about myself – when I am with people who want to be intimate with me?
☐ Can I confront others without trying to punish them, or do I play the game of I'm right – You're wrong?
☐ Do I ever talk to others about the strengths and weaknesses of our relationship?
☐ Do I make attempts to meet new people? Does the way in which I meet new people encourage them to make further contact with me?
☐ Am I an active listener – that is, do I both listen carefully and then respond to what I've heard?
☐ Do people I know come to me when they are in some kind of trouble? If they do, do they leave me feeling understood or helped?
☐ Am I outgoing, a go-getter in my relationships, or do I sit back and wait for others to make the first move?

Do I want to be very close to some people?

- What does closeness or intimacy mean to me? Does it mean deep conversations?   Does it mean touching and being physical?
- Do I enjoy it when others share with me whatever is important in their lives, including their secrets and deepest feelings?
- Do I like to share whatever is important in my life with others, including my secrets and deepest feelings?
- Which people am I close to now?
- Do I encourage certain others to get close to me? How do I encourage them to do this?
- Does closeness frighten me a bit? If so, what is it about closeness that frightens me?
- Are there many different ways of being close to others? What are these ways? Which ways do I prefer?

How do I handle my feelings and emotions when I am with others?

- Do others see me as a very feeling person, or do they see me a being rather cold and controlled?
- Which emotions do I express easily to others and which do I tend to wallow or hide?
- Is it easy for others to know what I am feeling?
- Do I let my emotions take over and rule me when I am with others?
- Do I try to control others by my emotions – for instance, by being moody, do I manipulate others?
- Do I think that it is right to be emotional with others?
- How do react when others are emotional towards me?
- Which emotions do I enjoy in others, which ones do I fear?
- What do I say when others keep their emotions locked up inside themselves?

How do I act when I feel I am being rejected by someone?

- Does feeling left out and being lonely play much of a part in my life?
- If I feel rejected how do I try to handle my feelings?

☐   Do I sometimes avoid getting to know someone, or joining a group of people, because I am afraid I will be rejected?

☐   Can other people scare me easily?

☐   Have I ever really been let down or rejected by someone?

☐   How easily am I hurt, and what do I do when I get hurt?

☐   Do I ignore or reject others who might want to get close to me?

Handout Five

Statements on My Interpersonal Style

1. Statement:
   a. I'm shy. My shyness takes the form of being afraid to meet new people and of being afraid to talk about myself deeply with the friends I do have.
   b. I am an outgoing person. I enjoy meeting new people. I even look for opportunities to get to know people.

2. Statement:
   a. I don't push myself enough in interpersonal situations. Others can step on me and I usually take it without saying much.
   b. I stand up for my rights fairly well. I am kind to others, but I don't let them step on me or control me.

3. Statement:
   a. I get angry very easily, and I dump my anger on others freely. I often get angry because I don't get my own way.
   b. Although I become angry at times, I do not lose control. When I am angry with someone, I tell the person so and try to settle what is bothering me

4. Statement:
   a. I am a lone person. I find it especially hard to take the time and energy needed to get to know others.
   b. I'm a very energetic person. I like listening to and getting involved with others. I work hard at the relationships I have.

5. Statement:
   a. I'm somewhat fearful of persons of the opposite sex, especially if I get the feeling that they want some kind of special closeness with me.
   b. I get along very well with persons of the opposite sex and I can have many different kinds of relationships with them, from casual friends to someone very close.

6. Statement:
   a. I am not a very sensitive person. I find it hard to know what others are feeling and often I don't care.
   b. I am usually aware of what others are feeling. Often I find myself experiencing something of the same emotion as someone else, just by listening to them.

7. Statement:
   a. I have too much self-control. I ordinarily don't let my emotions show at all. Sometimes I think that I would rather not have emotions at all.
   b. I express my emotions well. I don't dump them on others, but I don't try to hide them either. Others usually know what I am feeling.

8. Statement:
   a. I like to control others. But I don't want others to know that I am doing it. In my relationships I want to be the person in charge.
   b. There is a great deal of give and take in my relationships with others, I don't let them boss me around, but I don't have to be the person in charge either.

9. Statement:
   a. I have a very strong need to be liked by others. I want everyone I meet to like me. I seldom do anything that will offend anyone.
   b. I like to be liked by others, but that isn't the most important thing in my life. I want to do what I think is right, even if others don't like it. I don't like to offend others, but I don't need everyone's approval either.

10. Statement:
   a. I feel that I just have to help others. I get nervous when I am not doing something for someone else.
   b. Helping others is important, but it's also important for me to have time for myself. I don't need people who need my help or who want me to do favours for them in order for me to feel good about myself.

11. Statement:
    a. I'm very easily hurt. I send out messages to others that say be careful of me.
    b. I don't keep thinking that others might hurt me. I roll with the punches pretty well. I can laugh at myself. Others know they can be loose when they are around me.

12. Statement:
    a. I don't want to be dependent, so I fight others. I always have to show that I am free and a person in my own right. I find it quite difficult to get along with people in authority.
    b. I like co-operating and working with others. I can influence others and let others influence me. I can depend on others and let them depend on me in a good sense.

13. Statement:
    a. I'm an anxious person, especially in interpersonal situations. I don't know why I am like that.
    b. I'm a relaxed person, although I do get anxious at times, it's more like me to be relaxed in interpersonal situations.

14. Statement:
    a. I am a somewhat colourless and uninteresting person. I have a few interests. I am bored with myself at times and I assume others are bored with me.
    b. I am a colourful and interesting person, others enjoy being with me. I add life and excitement at gatherings, and I like this part of myself very much.

15. Statement:
    a. I take too many risks and I am too daring in interpersonal situations. I am impulsive, I lack self-control.
    b. I take reasonable risks in interpersonal situations. I have fairly good self control.

16. Statement:
    a. I'm very stubborn. I think my opinions are more important than anyone else's opinion. I am ready to argue with anyone at any time.
    b. I have an open mind. While I have ideas of my own, I don't go around looking for arguments. I enjoy sharing my opinions with others and can even change my opinions when I see something better.

17. Statement:
    a. I'm a rather sneaky person. I seduce people in various ways (not necessarily sexual ones). I get them to do what I want.
    b. I'm open and direct in my relationships with others. If I want anything from anyone, I ask them for it as plainly as possible. I am not sneaky or seductive.

18. Statement:
    a. I'm a selfish person I usually put my own needs and comforts before the needs of others.
    b. I can be generous when I want. There are times when I do put the needs of others before my needs and comfort.

19. Statement:
    a. I feel awkward when I am with people. I don't do the right things at the right time. I don't notice when others are having a rough time.
    b. I am very much at home with people. I'm sensitive to what those around me are feeling and I usually respond to what they are feeling in a human way. I usually know the right thing to do at the right time.

20. Statement:
    a. I am rather lonely. I don't think that others really like me, I spend a lot of time feeling sorry for myself.
    b. I experience loneliness from time to time, but it is not a big thing. I know that people think that I am alright. I don't spend much time feeling sorry for myself.

21. Statement:
    a. I am stingy. I don't share my time or money very easily.
    b. I'm a generous person. I like to share what I have with others, and I like to receive what others have to share with me.

22. Statement:
    a. I have lived a too sheltered a live. I feel out of it; I don't really know the score on life. Others have had many more experiences than I have had. They know life a lot better.
    b. I've had plenty of human experiences. I know the score just as well as the next person. I'm not just a kid.

23. Statement:
    a. I'm something of a coward. I find it hard to stand up for my opinions and convictions. It is easy to get me to retreat.
    b. I have the courage of my convictions. It is not easy to baby me. I know what my values are and can stand fast with them even when others challenge me.

24. Statement:
    a. When I am challenged or confronted, I tend to run away or attack the person confronting me. I get scared.
    b. When I am confronted, I listen to what the other person has to say. I try to make sure I understand what he or she says. I try to respond without being defensive.

Handout Six

Maslow's Characteristics of Self-actualized People

A. Priority of Values like Truth, Love, and Happiness

☐ **Acceptance of self, of others, of nature:** 'not complaining about water because it is wet', stoic style of calmly accepting even the worst.

☐ **Identification with the human species:** identification with all of humanity versus just their own family, friends, culture, or nation.

☐ **Emphasis on higher level values:** (see Handout Seven)

☐ **Perception of reality:** greater perceptual accuracy of reality, superior ability to reason and perceive the truth, and understand people at a deeper level.

☐ **Discrimination between means and ends, between good and evil:** clearer and more focused upon ends than most people, although they view their experiences and activities more as ends in themselves than most people.

☐ **Resolution of dichotomies (conflicts):** resolve conflicts that plague most people, because of their highly developed, accepting philosophy of life.

B. Internally Controlled

☐ **Autonomy and resistance to enculturation:** nonconformity. Not susceptible to social pressure to 'fit in'.

☐ **Detachment and desire for privacy:** high enjoyment of privacy and solitude. Calm and at peace with themselves.

☐ **Spontaneity, simplicity, naturalness:** reflects integration of values and habits. Open, integrated values and habits.

C. High Involvement, Productivity, and Happiness

☐ **Problem-centring:** easily forgets self and easily absorbed in tasks they love and/or feel are extremely important.

☐ **Creativeness:** retain an almost childlike, fresh, naive, and direct way of looking at life. Maybe partly the result of other factors such as problem-centring.

☐ **Freshness of appreciation and richness of emotional reactions:** ability to intensely focus on the present and highly involved in it. Very accepting of emotions.

☐ **High frequency of peak experiences:** sudden feelings of intense joy, happiness, and well-being. More at one with yourself and the world, more integrated, interconnected, and in harmony.

D. High-quality Interpersonal Relationships

☐ **(Intimate) interpersonal relations:** deeper and more profound interpersonal relations than any other adults. However, these very close relationships are often limited to a very few people. They tend to be kind, affectionate, friendly, and unpretentious, but can be direct and assertive when needed.

☐ **Democratic character structure:** a person's status is unimportant to them.

☐ **Philosophical, unhostile sense of humour.**

(The above describes the growth process from a lower to a higher level of functioning).

Handout Seven

Maslow's Metavalues (or 'Being' Values)

Focusing on satisfying the following values is important, and is why self-actualized people are happier, more peaceful, and more productive than other people. Self-actualized people have learned to look at life on a broader level. They are attentive to deadlines, getting jobs, relationships, and so on, but are not carried away, preoccupied, by them. Consequently they are not so emotionally affected by the ups and downs of daily life. They feel a sense of happiness from seeing progress towards satisfying these stable inner values (listed below) that do not depend so much upon external conditions. (www.csulb.edu)

- ☐ Wholeness (unity, integration, organization, simplicity)
- ☐ Perfection
- ☐ Completion
- ☐ Justice
- ☐ Aliveness (process, life, spontaneity, self-regulation, versus over-controlled)
- ☐ Richness (differentiation, complexity, intricacy)
- ☐ Simplicity
- ☐ Beauty
- ☐ Goodness
- ☐ Uniqueness (idiosyncrasy, individuality, novelty)
- ☐ Effortlessness (ease, grace, beautifully functioning)
- ☐ Playfulness (fun, joy, amusement, humour)
- ☐ Truth
- ☐ Self-sufficiency (autonomy, taking care of oneself)

When a self-actualizing person's values are threatened they do not tend to regress back to the earlier phase of development, instead their higher values are still more important them, once established higher values become very resistant to deterioration. Self-actualizing people spend less time with people or groups who do not share or emphasise these values. They also increase their understanding and care of others.

Handout Eight

Trait Checklist

It is suggested that you move quickly through the following list of traits. Use a tick beside those that you believe fits your self-image. Use an X to mark those that do not fit. Use a question mark in order to indicate the ones you are unsure about.

like myself

afraid of, or hurt by others

people can trust me

put up a good front

usually say the right thing

feel bad about myself

fearful of the future

dependent on others

waste time

use my talents

think for myself

don't understand myself

feel hemmed in

use time well

people avoid me

disinterested in community problems

enjoy work

enjoy nature

don't enjoy work

can't hold a job

trust myself

usually say the wrong thing

enjoy people

don't enjoy being the sex I am

discouraged about life

don't like to be around people

have not developed my talents

glad I'm the sex I am

often do the wrong thing

involved in solving community problems

people like to be around me

competent on the job

control myself

enjoy life

don't like myself

trouble controlling myself

Now look at the traits you have marked. Is there a pattern? Are they positive traits, negative, or a mixture? What traits would you like to change?

Handout Nine

Considering My Script and Other Questions

☐ Does your name or the names of either of your parent's names mean anything special in your family?

☐ Which family members do you get along with best?

☐ What are your favourite TV shows?

☐ What magazines or newspapers do you read?

☐ Who are your favourite entertainers?

☐ What kind of person are you?

☐ What kind of people are your mother and father?

☐ Did any other adults live in your home before you were 10 years old?

☐ What were you mother's and your father's favourite saying/s about life?

☐ How did your mother and your father praise you, what did they each say?

☐ How did your mother and your father criticise you, what did they each says?

☐ When your mother, and when your father were upset how did they each show it?

☐ What is your mother's advice to you, and what is your father's advice to you?

☐ How would your mother and how would your father describe you at aged five, and now?

☐ What nicknames have you had and what do they mean?

☐ What did your mother and what did your father hope you would be?

- What do you like most about yourself?
- What do you dislike most about yourself?
- What fairy tale or story did you like as child?
- What person did you like best and what did you like about the person?
- Who is a person you admire?
- What is the best thing you can do with your life?
- What is the worst thing you can do with your life?
- At what age have you thought you would die and how would your death occur?
- What feelings or thoughts are not allowed in your home?
- What will you do if things get really bad in your life?
- If things keep happening the way they are now, where will you be in five years from now?
- What happens to people like you?
- How do you see the world?
- What do you want most from your studies?

Handout Ten

Exploring Thoughts and Feelings

This exercise, which begins to explore your own self-concept, is not about evaluating you but rather an exercise to help you know more about yourself. It may also assist you in exploring issues which may ultimately be of help to you.

Think about each of the statements and decide if you own them as being definitely not true, tends to be true, is especially true. As you go through the process particular statements may hold a particular relevance for you and therefore suggest further work.

☐ I am important

☐ I feel warmth towards myself

☐ I am a significant individual

☐ I don't feel I can rely upon my own judgement

☐ I feel affectionate towards myself

☐ I feel like an important person

☐ I like myself

☐ I feel personally distant from myself

☐ I trust my own abilities

☐ I feel very friendly towards myself

☐ I am suspicious of my own competence

☐ I think that I am an interesting person

☐ I trust my own competence

☐ I feel that I am an intriguing person

☐ I have confidence in my own abilities

☐ I am a stimulating person

☐ I can depend on my own judgement

☐ I hate myself

Handout Eleven

Further Exploration of Self

Complete the following sentences, and then go back and tick the ones you think are most significant for you. This exercise is extremely valuable in terms of self-disclosure, and for getting beyond the surface; issues arising can be used for further work on a one to one basis or within the study group.

- ☐ People who love me...
- ☐ One thing I really like about myself is...
- ☐ I dislike people who...
- ☐ When people ignore me...
- ☐ The way I am generous with others is...
- ☐ When someone praises me...
- ☐ When I relate to people, I...
- ☐ When I relate to people they...
- ☐ Those who really know me...
- ☐ When I let someone know something I don't like about myself...
- ☐ My mother...
- ☐ My moods when I am with others...
- ☐ I am at my best with people when...
- ☐ When I am in a group of strangers...
- ☐ I feel lonely when...
- ☐ I envy...
- ☐ When someone is affectionate with me...
- ☐ When I take a good look at my interpersonal relationships I,
- ☐ The way I handle jealousy is...
- ☐ I think I've hurt others by...
- ☐ Those who don't know me well...
- ☐ My brother...
- ☐ The person who knows me best...
- ☐ An important person of value for me is...
- ☐ What I'm really looking for in my relationship is...
- ☐ I get hurt when...
- ☐ I daydream about...
- ☐ My family...
- ☐ When someone confronts me...

- What I feel most guilty about in my relationship with others is...
- I am at my worst with people when...
- I like people who...
- When someone gets angry with me...
- My sister...
- Few people know that I...
- I think about closeness, I think about...
- When I meet someone who is very strong and outgoing...
- When I don't like someone who likes me I...
- When I am not around my friends...
- Most people think that I...
- One thing I really dislike about myself is...
- When I am with a group of my friends...
- I get angry when someone...
- What I distrust most in others is...
- One thing that makes me nervous in interpersonal situations is...
- When I really feel good about myself I...
- When others put me down...
- In relation to others, I get a big lift when...
- In my interpersonal relationships this year I learned that...
- When I like someone who doesn't like me I...
- I feel awkward and out of place with others when...
- When others act like my parents towards me I...
- The thing that holds me back in my relationships with others is...
- Too many people...
- When I share my values with someone...
- I would like the person I want as a partner...
- Others like it when I...
- Interpersonal relationships are important but...
- When others see the ways in which I can be hurt...
- In interpersonal situations what I run away from most is...

Bibliography

Allport GW (1937)   **Personality: A Psychological Interpretation,** New York: Rinehart & Winston Inc.

Berne E (1964)   **Games People Play,** Harmondsworth: Penguin Books.

Berne E (1976)   **Beyond Games and Scripts,** New York: Grove Press.

Biestek FP (1961)   **Casework Relationship,** London: George Allen and Inwin Limited.

Bion WR (1961)   **Experiences in Groups and Other Papers** London: Tavistock Press

Davison G, Neal J (1974)   **Abnormal Psychology,** New York: Wiley & Son Inc.

Dewey J (1933)   **How We Think,** Boston: Heath & Co. Inc.

Egan G (1975)   **The Skilled Helper,** Brooks Cole: California.

Elliot R   **Revised Session Reactions Scale:** www.experiential-researchers.org

Eysenk HJ (1954)   **The Psychology of Politics,** London: Routledge, Kegan Paul.

Frankel VE (1959)   **Man's Search for Meaning,** London: Hogarth Press.

Freud S (1920)   **Beyond the Pleasure Principle**, Vol. 18, London: Hogarth Press.

Harris TA (1967)   **I'm OK, You're OK,** London: Johnathan Cape.

James M, Jongeward D (1978)   **Born To Win,** New York, New York: Signet Classics.

Jersild AT (1952)   **In Search of Self,** New York: Bureaux Publications.

Jongeward D, Seyer P (1978)   **Choosing Success: Transactional Analysis on the Job,** New York: John Wiley & Sons, Inc.

Jung C G (1986)	**The Collective Works, Archetypes, and the Collective Unconscious**, London: Routledge.
Knight R (1984)	**(Chapter in) Management in the Special School,** London: Croom Helm.
Knight R (2010)	**Colon Hydrotherapy: The Professional Practitioner Training Manual and Reference Book**, Chelmsford: Cross Roads Publications.
Knight R (2004)	**How to Practise Complementary Medicine Professionally,** Bury St Edmunds: Arima.
Klein M (1963)	**Our Adult World and Other Essays,** London: Heinemann.
Kopp S (1974)	**An End to Innocence,** London: Sheldon Press.
Laing RD (1971)	**The Politics of the Family,** London: Tavistock Publications.
Maslow AH (1971)	**Self-actualizing and Beyond, The Farther Reaches of Human Nature, New York:** The Viking Press.
Munro A et al. (1989)	**Counselling: The Skills of Problem Solving,** London: Routledge.
Nelson-Jones R (1990)	**Practical Counselling and Helping Skills**, London: Cassell.
Roger CR (1961)	**On Becoming a Person,** Boston: Houghton Miffin Company.
Roger CR (1951)	**Client-Centred Therapy,** Boston: Houghton Miffin Company.
Schiff JL (1975)	**Cathexis Reader,** New York: Harper and Roe.
Steiner CM (1980)	**Scripts People Live,** New York: Grove Press.
Woollams S, Brown M (1979)	**The Total Handbook of Transactional Analysis,** Englewood Cliffs: Prentice Hall.

Index

178

179

R

S

T

184

About the Author

Richard has worked in the helping professions for over 45 years as a practitioner, therapist, teacher, manager, trainer, lecturer, consultant, and in research and development. He holds professional qualifications in child care, education, art therapy, nutrition, and colon hydrotherapy. His doctorate is in psychotherapy and counselling.

Richard has run training courses nationally for central government departments and other organisations, on the care, treatment, and appropriate therapeutic interventions for emotionally disturbed children and adults. He studied Transactional Analysis at the Cathexis Institute in California and Oregon State Hospital. Richard is a Fellow of the Association of Natural Medicine and a Fellow of the Royal Society of Arts.

Books by the same author:

Colon Hydrotherapy: The Professional Practitioner Training Manual and Reference Book: Cross Roads Publications (2010).

How to Practise Complementary Medicine Professionally:
Arima Publishing (Third Edition 2004).

Notes

Notes

Notes

Lightning Source UK Ltd.
Milton Keynes UK
08 April 2011

170569UK00001B/8/P